Depression Research in Nursing

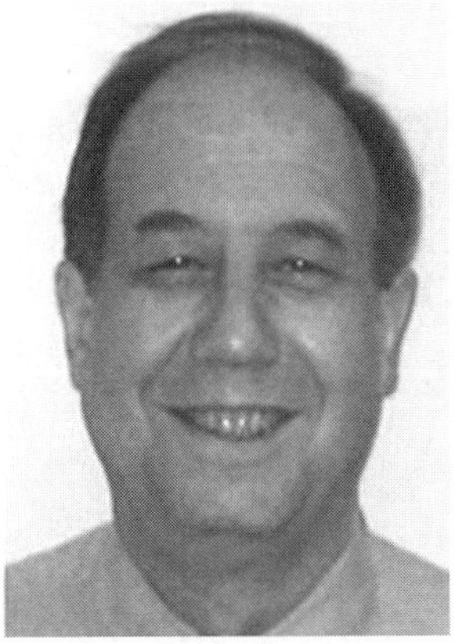

Reg Arthur Williams, PhD, RN, CS, FAAN, is a Professor at the School of Nursing and at the Department of Psychiatry, Medical School, the University of Michigan. He is a Fellow of the American Academy of Nursing. His research and writing are in the areas of depression, stress, and coping. He also carries a caseload of individuals with depression through the Depression Center at the University of Michigan. Dr. Williams holds a Master's in Nursing in psychosocial nursing and a PhD from University of Washington, Seattle, Washington.

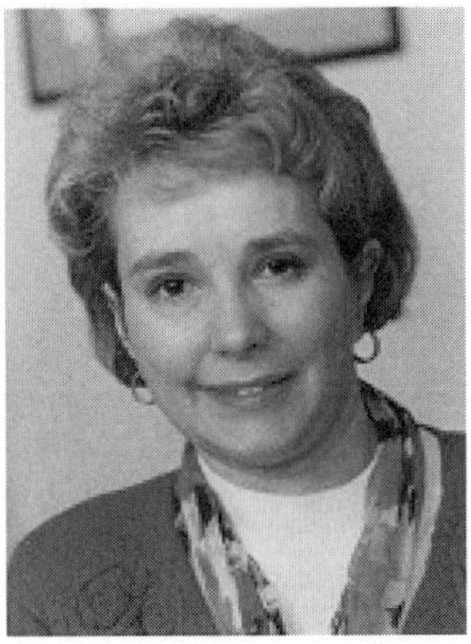

Bonnie M. Hagerty, PhD, RN, CS, is an Associate Professor in the School of Nursing and an adjunct clinical nurse specialist at the Depression Center, the University of Michigan. Her research focuses on recurrent depression, including prodromal symptoms of recurrence, self-management, and adherence to antidepressants. She is a coinvestigator with Dr. Reg Williams on projects related to depression in U.S. Navy recruits and the effectiveness of a specific cognitive-behavioral intervention. Dr. Hagerty developed the theory of Human Relatedness and has examined the concept of sense of belonging. Her Sense of Belonging Instrument is used worldwide. Dr. Hagerty received her BS in Nursing from Russell Sage College in Troy, New York. She completed her MS in Nursing at the University of Maryland and a joint PhD in Nursing and Higher Education at the University of Michigan.

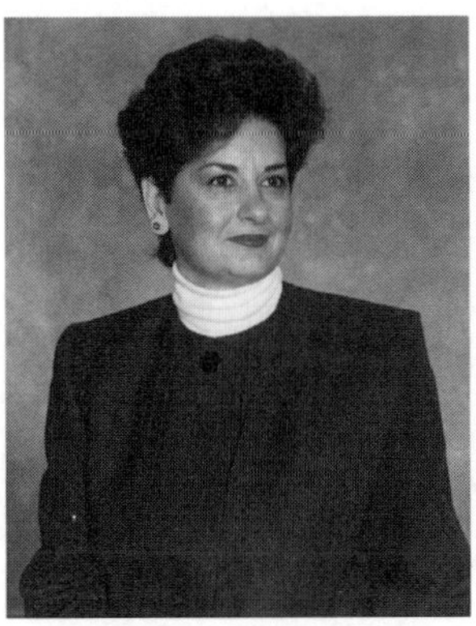

Shaké Ketefian, EdD, RN, FAAN, is Professor and Director of International Affairs at the University of Michigan School of Nursing, Ann Arbor, Michigan, and is a Fellow of the American Academy of Nursing. Her research and writing have focused on application of research to practice and education, ethical issues in health care, scientific integrity, global issues in knowledge development, and international graduate and doctoral education. Dr. Ketefian is a cofounder and founding President of the International Network for Doctoral Education in Nursing. She served as the Editor of *Research and Theory for Nursing Practice: An International Journal*.

Depression Research in Nursing

GLOBAL PERSPECTIVES

Reg Arthur Williams & Bonnie Hagerty
VOLUME EDITORS

Shaké Ketefian
EXECUTIVE EDITOR

Springer Publishing Company

Springer Publishing Company, Inc.
11 West 42nd Street
New York, NY 10036

Acquisitions Editor: Ruth Chasek
Production Editor: Sara Yoo
Cover design by Mimi Flow

05 06 07 08 09/5 4 3 2 1

Library of Congress Cataloging-in-Publication Data

Depression research in nursing : global perspectives / Reg Arthur Williams, Bonnie Hagerty, volume editors ; Shaké Ketefian, executive editor.
p. ; cm.
Includes bibliographical references.
Summary: "This book focuses on depression research by nurses with individuals with intellectual and developmental disabilities, postpartum and prenatal depression, chronic illness, posttraumatic brain injury, and other illnesses"—Provided by publisher.
ISBN 0-8261-5765-3 (soft cover)
1. Depression, Mental—Nursing. 2. Depression, Mental—Complications—Nursing. 3. Psychiatric nursing.
[DNLM: 1. Depressive Disorder--complications. 2. Nursing Research. WM 171 D4241993 2005] I. Williams, Reg Arthur. II. Hagerty, Bonnie Kawczak. III. Ketefian, Shaké.

RC537.D4453 2005
616.85'27'0231—dc22 2005003750

Printed in the United States of America by Capital City Press.

Contents

Contributors

Sarah H. Ailey, PhD, RN
Rush University College of Nursing
Department of Community and Mental Health Nursing
Chicago, IL

Esther Bay, APRN, BC, PhD
Assistant Professor
Michigan State University
East Lansing, MI

Susan Brust, MS, RN, CNS, PsyNP
Clinical Nurse Specialist
Zumbro Valley Mental Health Center
Rochester, MN

Hsiu-Ju Chang, PhD, MSN, RN
Frances Payne Bolton School of Nursing
Case Western Reserve University
Cleveland, OH

Julia Muennich Cowell, PhD, RN, FAAN
Chair, Department of Community and Mental Health Nursing
College of Nursing
Rush University
Chicago, IL

Laila F. Farhood, PhD, RN, CS
American University of Beirut
School of Nursing
Riad El Solh
Beirut, Lebanon

Louis Fogg, PhD
Community and Mental Health Nursing
College of Nursing
Rush University
Chicago, IL

Carol Fristedt
Department of Nursing
Mayo Clinic
Rochester, MN

Brenda Gillespie, PhD
Assistant Professor, Center for Statistical Research
University of Michigan
Ann Arbor, MI

Janice Goodman, PhD, APRN, BC
William F. Connell School of Nursing
Boston College
Chestnut Hill, MA

Deborah Gross, DNSc, RN, FAAN
College of Nursing
Rush University
Chicago, IL

Barbara A. Hayes, RN, DNSc, FRCNA
Professor of Nursing, School of Nursing Sciences
James Cook University
Townsville, Australia

June Andrews Horowitz, PhD, APRN-BC, FAAN
William F. Connell School of Nursing
Boston College
Chestnut Hill, MA

Ned Kirsch, PhD
Adjunct Assistant Professor
Department of Psychology
University of Michigan
Ann Arbor, MI

Diane B. McNaughton. PhD, RN
Community and Mental Health Nursing
Rush University College of Nursing
Chicago, IL

Arlene Miller, PhD, RN, CS
Department Head, Public Health, Mental Health and Administrative Nursing
College of Nursing
University of Illinois at Chicago
Chicago, IL

Diana L. Morris, RN, PhD, FAAN
Associate Professor of Nursing and Associate Director, University Center on Aging and Health
Frances Payne Bolton School of Nursing
Case Western Reserve University
Cleveland, OH

Reinhold Muller, PhD, MSc
Associate Professor in Epidemiology and Biostatistics
School of Public Health and Tropical Medicine
James Cook University
Townsville, Australia

V. Shane Pankratz, PhD
Department of Health Sciences Research
Division of Biostatics
Mayo Clinic
Rochester, MN

Pamela Pierce, MS, CNP
Department of Nursing
Mayo Clinic
Rochester, MN

Sunida Preechawong, PhD, RN
Faculty of Nursing
Chulalongkorn University
Patumwan, Bangkok, Thailand

Sopin Sangon, PhD, RN
Psychiatric and Mental Health Unit
Department of Nursing
Ramathibodi Faculty of Medicine
Mahidol University
Rachathevee, Thailand

Sharon Tucker, DNSc, RN, CNS
Clinical Nurse Researcher/Nurse Administrator
Department of Nursing
Division of Nursing Research
Mayo Clinic
Rochester, MN

Jaclene A. Zauszniewski, PhD, RNC
Frances Payne Bolton School of Nursing
Case Western Reserve University
Cleveland, OH

Preface

Shaké Ketefian

Depression has become a major international health issue. With wars, mass displacements and migrations, large segments of the world's populations suffer from emotional and mental health disorders. Manifestations may vary in different parts of the world, given the particular circumstances communities face.

In view of this compelling health problem, the editors of this book, which originated as a special issue of the journal *Research and Theory for Nursing Practice: An International Journal,* determined that a volume on depression research would shed light on this and related phenomena, and assist clinicians in their practice. Drs. Reg Williams and Bonnie Hagerty are two outstanding nurse scholars whose program of research over the past decade has dealt with depression research. We are most grateful to them for serving as editors for this volume, and for the wisdom and expertise they brought to bear in the preparation of this project.

We collectively made every effort to include international perspectives in the preparation of this volume. In addition, the authors deal with special populations and multicultural groups in presenting their research.

1

Depression Research: Nursing's Contributions

Reg Arthur Williams
Bonnie Hagerty

The impact and burden of depression are profound. The problem of depression is worldwide. Murray and Lopez, using World Health Organization (WHO) data (Murray & Lopez, 1996), and Greden (2001) have noted that there are powerful epidemiological data demonstrating that depression is one of the most burdensome and disabling disorders in the world. WHO compared 100 diseases, and depression ranked fourth in global burden. As well, WHO projected that depression, as a global burden, will be ranked second by the year 2010 if prevention, diagnosis, and treatment do not have meaningful improvements. In addition, WHO ranked depression first with years lived with the disability and also first in women for worldwide burden. This was true for developed and developing countries alike.

In the United States, depression is a major public health concern (Murray & Lopez, 1996; U.S. Department of Health and Human Services [USDHHS], 2000), recognized by the Surgeon General as one of the top 10 health problems in the United States. *Healthy People 2010* (USDHHS, 2000) specifies the need for better recognition and treatment of depression as one of the critical health care goals over the next decade. Over 21% of women and 12% of men will experience an episode of major depression during their lifetime, and symptom onset is highest in the teens and early 20s (Kessler, Avenevoli, & Merikangas, 2001; Kessler et al., 1994). In fact, depression is the most common mental disorder in adolescence and is the forerunner of later recurrent and chronic illness (Patton, 1998).

The results of depression are devastating, causing suffering and anguish for individuals, families, friends, and communities. Families and employers expend both personal and economic resources to deal with the persons' depression and depressive symptoms. A major concern is that early depression signals a future recurrent or chronic depression that becomes increasingly debilitating (Greden, 2001).

Depression, now recognized as a complex genetic disorder, may come about as a result of the interplay of genetic vulnerability and environmental triggers such as stress (Post, 1992; Williams, Hagerty, Yousha, Horrocks, Hoyle, & Liu, in press). Given a genetic predisposition to depression, life events may trigger the onset of depressive symptoms through activation of stress mechanisms (Kendler, Karkowski,

& Prescott, 1999). Factors that may predispose an individual to depression include female gender (Kessler et al., 1994; Nolen-Hoeksema, 1995), family history of mood disorders (Kendler, Thornton, & Gardner, 2001; Williams, Hagerty, Yousha, Hoyle, & Oe, 2002), personal history of depressive symptoms, abuse, and family conflict (Kendler, Gardner, & Prescott, 2002; Williams et al., 2002). The juxtaposition of factors such as an early onset, failure to recognize and properly treat the illness, and its eventual recurrent and damaging course, all point to the need for nursing research to examine strategies for people who suffer from depression and for its prevention.

HISTORY OF DEPRESSION AND ITS TREATMENT

As Ailey and Miller point out in the chapter in this volume, Hippocrates first wrote about the clinical description of depression in fourth century BC. Hippocrates thought depression was caused by excessive black bile *'melan chole'*; from which *melancholy* was derived. The term is still used today to usually denote severe depression. Even in those earliest times, depression was thought to be a physiological disorder. Yet by the time of the dark ages, people viewed mental illness as sinister or evil. Sinister religious reasons were often attributed as the cause of the illness. Even into the 20th century, the psychoanalytic view of the cause of depression was "the frustration of oral needs for love and gratification by a mothering figure" (Johnson, 1993, p. 439). Many psychosocial theories abounded, as outlined by Ailey and Miller.

It is only in the last 15 to 20 years that a beginning understanding has emerged regarding the complex brain mechanisms involved in depression. We now know that depression is a brain illness (Greden, 2001). It is treatable. There are more than 40 antidepressants on the market and many more in development and testing phases. We know that by combining therapy (often cognitive/behavioral approaches) and medication effectively, more than 85% of people suffering from depression are helped.

Despite these advances in treatment for depression, only about 10% to 15% of the total population of depressed people receive adequate treatment (Greden, 2001). The stigma of depression remains profound. Individuals are reluctant to seek evaluation and treatment because they fear they might jeopardize their job, their status with their family and friends, or their own image, or because they deem the costs of treatment too high. Too many still hold the image of treatment as described by Kesey (1962) in *One Flew Over the Cuckoo's Nest*, with the use of electro-convulsive therapy. Today's treatments are dramatically different and more effective than what was depicted by Kesey.

In response to the overwhelming need for meaningful improvements in prevention, diagnosis, treatment, and research on depression, the University of Michigan established the first comprehensive Depression Center in the United States in 2001. The Center uses a multidisciplinary approach to depression; therefore, behavioral scientists, neuroscientists, clinical investigators, nurse researchers, specialty physicians, student health providers, nurses, and primary care physicians work together to deliver quality care to patients and their families. One goal of the Depression Center is to diminish the stigma of depression. Greden has pointed out "other disorders, like cancer, were stigmatized in the past. Now, we have a national network of 21 cancer centers. Ten years from now, I hope we will have a national network of depression centers and it is our goal to make Michigan a prototype" (2002, p. 25).

DEPRESSION RESEARCH IN NURSING

Depression has finally captured the attention of not only mental health providers, but also those in other medical specialties and health-related professions, as well as persons involved in public policy. Depression is a recurrent, chronic illness that requires care for acute episodes as well as management of the illness over time. Psychiatry has focused on treatment of the illness and symptom management of acute episodes. Psychiatrists have paid minimal attention to the person's response to the illness, issues arising from the interaction between the person and environment, or concerns over patients' management of the illness within the context of their lives. Therefore, nursing is in a unique position to generate new knowledge about depression, people's responses to depression, and its associated phenomena.

Nurse researchers have studied depression using a variety of perspectives and study designs. Qualitative studies have explored the life experiences of people with depression. Quantitative research has been correlational or predictive, examining factors and characteristics associated with depression. Depression has been an outcome variable as well as a predictor variable in these correlational studies. In addition, nurse researchers have conducted intervention studies in which the effectiveness of specific interventions was determined.

In many nursing studies, the focus of the research has been on another concept relevant to depression such as caregiving, loneliness, and sense of belonging. In these studies, depression is considered a correlate, predictor, or an intervening variable in relationship to the concept being studied. Thus, we see how depression contributes to and is associated with other phenomena.

Many of the nursing studies use the term "depression" broadly, without clear conceptual definitions. Depression has been examined as a mood, a component of grief, a collection of depressive symptoms, and an acute and chronic illness based on established diagnostic criteria. Each of these conceptualizations of depression implies differences in expression of symptoms, clinical course, and interventions. As a result, nursing research on depression tends to be fragmented with no one conceptual focus. Also, there is minimal evidence that results from nursing research on depression have been incorporated into clinical practice. Extensive work on depression is required. Qualitative studies can help us understand people's experience of depression, which should help nurses understand and work with persons with depression. We need quantitative research to determine phenomena that are related to depression and how to best intervene. Nursing research that guides our understanding and approach to persons with depression is essential.

There are multiple perspectives from which to examine depression, such as biological, interpersonal, and psychological models. Yet there has been little research in nursing or in other fields about how people cope with depression as a chronic, recurrent illness. For example, although we have evidence that depression is manifested differently by characteristics such as gender, race, and culture, we know very little about the mechanisms, both biological and sociocultural, that create or contribute to these differences, or the different treatment approaches appropriate for different patient groups.

Over the past decade there has been important research on the relationship of depression to other illnesses such as cardiovascular disease (Sullivan, LaCroix, Spectus, & Hecht, 2000). It appears that depression may affect the development of other illnesses and influence health outcomes just as other illnesses may contribute to depression. For example, there is evidence that persons with depression have a higher mortality from cardiovascular disease than those without depression (Barefoot, et al., Helms, Mark, Blumenthal, Califf, & Haney, 1996). The chapter by Bay and colleagues contributes to this area of inquiry by examining stress and depression after traumatic brain injury (TBI). Remarkably, little research exists about depression and TBI, and Bay's study provides new knowledge about this important topic.

One notable area of interest for research on depression has focused on postnatal depression. Sadly, both health care researchers and the public have attended to prenatal depression only recently, as a result of recent high-profile cases in which women with postpartum depression have killed their children. Nurse researchers have investigated prenatal and postpartum depression to better understand how to assess women for prenatal depression and how best to intervene. Contributors to this volume, Horowitz and Goodman, investigate women's postpartum depression over a 2-year period. Based on their longitudinal study, the authors report results that can influence the assessment of women's postpartum depression over time rather than just weeks after delivery. Hayes and Muller discuss the results of their study of pre- and postnatal depression. Their findings provide empirical support for different profiles of prenatal and postpartum depression, data that can guide nurses in earlier assessment of depression in pregnant women earlier in the pregnancy. These authors also describe testing the effect of an educational intervention on prenatal depression.

As mentioned earlier, depression is an international health problem, influenced by factors such as war, poverty, violence, and culture. Farhood's examination of stress in Lebanese families attends to the influence of war and disruptions in the environment, how families adapt and cope in difficult circumstances, and how various factors influence depression and its severity. For many cultures, little is known about how specific ethnic, racial, societal, and cultural factors influence the expression of depression and subsequent intervention. Sangon describes predictors of depression in Thai women, making a significant contribution to knowledge about women's depression in Thailand.

In addition to culture, depression occurs within the context of families and systems. Families can contribute to stress and, ultimately, depression in those individuals who are genetically vulnerable. In turn, the depressed person's behavior and negativity generate reactions from family members such as anger, avoidance, and guilt. The emotional tone and depressive behaviors within the family affect the children. McNaughton, Cowell, Gross, Fogg, and Ailey examine the relationship between child and maternal mental health in families who had emigrated from Mexico. Their findings demonstrate the extent to which depression is a problem for both mothers and their children. The study of this immigrant group of Mexican mothers and their children is an especially welcome addition to the literature, given the scarcity of studies on this and other ethnic groups who present unique challenges to the health care system.

Depression traverses the life span from childhood to adulthood to old age. Assessment of depression in the elderly has been neglected over the years. With aging baby boomers and rising health care costs, there has been increased attention to diagnosing and treating depression in the elderly. Assessing elders for depression can be problematic since some symptoms of depression, such as sleep difficulty, may not be pathological in older adults. Zauszniewski, Morris, Preechawong, and Chang examine the utility of three different instruments to assess elderly persons for depression. Their findings reinforce the importance of using multiple strategies to determine if an older person is depressed.

Ultimately, our goal is to intervene in a way that helps the depressed person attain health or manage the condition. This might be accomplished with specific therapeutic regimens initiated by the mental health providers or with strategies initiated by the person with depression. Describing self-efficacy as the confidence patients have that they can do what is necessary to control their illness, Tucker, Brust, Pierce, Fristedt, and Pankratz describe the results of a 2-year study on management of depression over time. This is particularly relevant given our understanding of the recurrent and chronic nature of this illness.

The chapters in this volume provide new knowledge about depression that can be translated into clinical care on both the individual and community levels. Depression should be a concern of every nurse, regardless of specialty. For as much as we know about depression, there is much more to discover. While physicians focus on etiology and medical treatment, nurse researchers must attend to how people express and deal with this crippling illness. We hope this volume ignites the readers' interest about depression for nursing research and for clinical practice.

REFERENCES

Barefoot, J. C., Helms, M. J., Mark, D. B., Blumenthal, J. A., Califf, R. M., Haney, T. L., et al. (1996). Depression and long-term mortality risk in patients with coronary artery disease. *American Journal of Cardiology, 78*, 613-617.

Greden, J. F. (Ed.). (2001). *Treatment of recurrent depression*. Washington, DC: American Psychiatric Publishing.

Greden, J. F. (2002). Conquering depression. *Medicine at Michigan, 4*, 20-29.

Johnson, B. S. (1993). *Psychiatric-mental health nursing: Adaptation and growth*. Philadelphia: Lippincott.

Kendler, K. S., Karkowski, L. M., & Prescott, C. A. (1999). Causal relationship between stressful life events and the onset of major depression. *American Journal of Psychiatry, 156*, 837-841.

Kendler, K. S., Thornton, L. M., & Gardner, C. O. (2001). Genetic risk, number of previous depressive episodes, and stressful life events in predicting onset of major depression. *American Journal of Psychiatry, 158*, 582-586.

Kendler, K. S., Gardner, C. O., & Prescott, C. A. (2002). Toward a comprehensive developmental model for major depression in women. *American Journal of Psychiatry, 159*, 1133-1145.

Kesey, K. (1962). *One flew over the cuckoo's nest*. New York: Viking Press.

Kessler, R. C., Avenevoli, S., & Merikangas, K. R. (2001). Mood disorders in children and adolescents: An epidemiologic perspective. *Biological Psychiatry, 49*, 1002–1014.

Kessler, R. C., McGonagle, K., Zhao, S., Nelson, C., Hughes, M., Eshleman, S., Wittchen, H., & Kendler, K. (1994). Lifetime and 12-month prevalence of DSM-III-R psychiatric disorders in the United States: Results from the national comorbidity survey. *Archives of General Psychiatry, 51*, 8-19.

McEwen, B. S. (2000). Effects of adverse experiences for brain structure and function. *Biological Psychiatry, 48*, 721-731.

Murray, C. J. L., & Lopez, A. D. (1996). Alternative visions of the future: Projecting mortality and disability, 1990-2020. In C. J. L. Murray & A. D. Lopez (Eds.), *The global burden of disease*. Boston: Harvard University Press.

Nolen-Hoeksema, S. (1995). Gender differences in coping with depression across the life span. *Depression*, 3, 81-90.

Patton, G. (1998). Adolescent psychiatry: Its potential to reduce the burden of mental disorder. *European Archives of Psychiatry and Clinical Neuroscience, 248*, 1-3.

Post, R. M. (1992). Transduction of psychosocial stress in the neurobiology of recurrent affective disorder. *American Journal of Psychiatry, 149*, 999-1010.

U.S. Department of Health and Human Services. (2000). *Healthy People 2010*. Washington, DC: U.S. Government Printing Office.

Sullivan, M. D., LaCroix, A. Z., Spectus, J. A., & Hecht, J. (2000). Five-year prospective study of the effects of anxiety and depression in patients with coronary artery disease. *American Journal of Cardiology, 86*, 1135-1138.

Williams, R. A., Hagerty, B. K., Yousha, S., Horrocks, J., Hoyle, K., & Liu, D. (in press). Psychosocial effects of the BOOT STRAP Intervention with Navy recruits. *Military Medicine*.

Williams, R. A., Hagerty, B. K., Yousha, S., Hoyle, K., & Oe, H. (2002). Factors associated with the onset of depression in Navy recruits. *Journal of Clinical Psychology, 58*(4), 323-337.

2

Psychosocial Theories of Depression for Individuals With Intellectual and Developmental Disabilities: A Historicist Perspective

Sarah H. Ailey
Arlene Miller

Depression is a major mental health problem, affecting about 15% to 17% of adults in the United States at some time in their lives (Kessler et al., 2003). A report from the Centers for Disease Control (CDC, 1996) estimates that about 1.5 million individuals in the United States have intellectual and developmental disabilities (I/DD). Depression is thought to be more common among individuals with I/DD than the general population (Borthwick-Duffy, 1994). Further, depression among individuals with I/DD is associated with poor outcomes, such as low levels of social support (Meins, 1993), social skills deficits (Matson, Smiroldo, Brandi, & Bamburg, 1998), and aggressive behavior and conduct problems (Meins, 1993; Reiss & Rojahn, 1993). Depression may hamper the ability of individuals with I/DD to take advantage of work, housing, and social opportunities and deserves to be treated adequately as part of preventing barriers to as full a participation in society as possible.

Depression has both biological and psychosocial aspects. The features of depression were recognized in ancient times. Beck (1967) notes that Hippocrates wrote the first clinical description of "melancholia" in the fourth century BC and that "there are few psychiatric syndromes whose clinical descriptions are so constant through successive eras of history" (p. 5). Jelliffe (1931), in a classic discussion of history, notes that descriptions of "melancholia" as a mood exist in the earliest records. Arataeus, a physician of the second century AD, wrote regarding "melancholia":

> The following are some of the more evident marks of the affection: the patients are quiet or sad, dejected and dull without any reason. . . . If it still comes to a greater height, they hate and shun society, complain of things the most trivial, curse life and covet

> death, the mind likewise of many border upon a state of total insensibility and infatuation, in so much as they are ignorant of everything, forgetful of themselves, and lead the life of beasts. (as cited in Jelliffe, 1931, pp. 369–370)

The descriptions of the ancients such as Arateus have similarity to current clinical descriptions of depression (American Psychiatric Association, 2000).

Theories regarding the psychosocial aspects of depression engender discussion and debate. In the last century there are four main groups of theories regarding the psychosocial aspects of depression: psychodynamic/psychoanalytic, behavioral, cognitive, and ecological/interpersonal theories (Clark, Beck, & Alford, 1999; Joiner, Coyne, & Blalock, 1999). These key groups of theories contain different views about human nature and the psychosocial aspects of depression and reflect the history of the times when they were developed.

Marginalization is a socio-political process that leads to groups of people being peripheral to the dominant society "on the basis of their identities, associations, experiences and environments" (Hall, Stevens, & Meleis, 1994, p. 25). Hall and colleagues note that marginalization is more inclusive than related processes such as oppression, alienation, and stigmatization. The concept of marginalization includes boundary maintenance dynamics and incorporates aspects of experience that are more inclusive than power imbalances and the subjective experiences of alienation and stigmatization. Marginalized groups are vulnerable to many health risks.

The history of individuals with I/DD in the US exposes how marginalization and oppression have both influenced science and have been influenced by science (Trent, 1994). For example, in the early 1900s, fear of individuals with I/DD was promoted and was involved in the development of eugenics as a "scientific" theory. Eugenics was widely discussed and applied to individuals with I/DD, being one of the rationales for the practices of large-scale institutionalization and forced sterilization (Trent, 1994), certainly practices that kept individuals with I/DD on the boundaries of society. Institutionalization of individuals with I/DD continued as the norm in the United States until the 1970s and individuals with I/DD were denied the right to live with their families and to have equal public education.

The marginalization of individuals with I/DD is also evident in the mental health care system. Until the mid-1980s, clinicians often thought that individuals with I/DD were not capable of depression (Sovner & Pary, 1993), characterizing them as too psychologically immature and worry-free to be depressed (Gardner, 1967). Individuals with I/DD continue to exist on the periphery of the mental health care system, with few practitioners receiving training regarding the specific mental health needs of the population (Szymanski & King, 1999).

Kessler and colleagues (2003) note that mental health problems in the general population are often not treated or inadequately treated. While it is now generally recognized that individuals with I/DD do have depression, they too are often not treated or inappropriately and inadequately treated. Individuals with I/DD are frequently referred for mental health care because of behavior problems (Hurley,

Folstein, & Lam, 2003). Estimates of behavior disorder prevalence range to over 60% of individuals with I/DD (Deb & Bright, 2001). Unfortunately, behavior disturbance or challenging behavior and psychiatric illness are terms used interchangeably for this population (Einfeld & Aman, 1995), and individuals who have disorders not associated with behavior problems may not be treated. For example, Edelstein and Glenwick (2001) used a series of vignettes to assess how direct-care workers identify psychological disorders of adults with I/DD and their need for treatment. Direct-care workers were more likely to identify behavioral symptoms and need for treatment of aggressive disorders and psychosis than depression, and to identify a need for treatment of aggressive disorders and psychosis than depression. This finding was present even though diagnostic information about depression and other mental health disorders in the adults with I/DD was given to the direct-care workers. In addition, individuals with I/DD are often given psychoactive drugs for chemical restraint in the absence of sound clinical rationales regarding diagnosis and clinical symptoms (Matson et al., 2000).

It is the thesis of this chapter that marginalization affects the application of the key groups of theories of the psychosocial aspects of depression with individuals with I/DD. Many of the techniques based in behavioral theories are focused on special populations, including individuals with I/DD (Dowd, 2002). Behavioral theories are limited, however, in regard to providing conceptions for identification, treatment, and research of depression in this population, and have significant ethical limitations. Cognitive theories of depression are well established and widely used in research and treatment of depression in the general population, but have limited usage in this population. Interpersonal theories of depression are used in the general population and have many benefits, but are only now being investigated for use with individuals with I/DD (Ailey, 2002).

HISTORICIST PERSPECTIVE

In a classic article, Silva and Rothbart (1984) suggest that nurse scholars should be aware of the influence of the philosophy of science on the development of nursing theory. Whall and Hicks (2002) note that philosophy of science is little discussed in U.S. nursing, but that progress in nursing science over the last 20 years is likely congruent with the philosophical ideas of Laudan (1977) and others. Debates regarding the philosophy of science affect discussions about the nature of nursing as a science (Edwards, 1999), the approaches to knowledge development in nursing (Reed, 1995), and the nature of evidence in nursing scientific inquiry (Forbes et al., 1999). Two major schools of philosophical thought are logical empiricism and historicism (Papineau, 1996; Silva & Rothbart, 1984). A logical empiricist perspective views scientific progress in terms of empirical testing that either tends to uphold or disprove theories. As empirical testing continues, theories are modified or changed to take account of new knowledge. Historicism, while recognizing this aspect of theory development, assesses the influences of an historical era, including marginalization, on the patterns of reasoning, scientific theories, and the practices of scientists. According to Kuhn (1962), historicism asks new sorts of questions and views science not as a cumulative but as a developmental process.

Laudan (1977, 1996) is a theorist in the historicist tradition and developed the concept of research traditions. Research traditions are a broadly based foundation of many theories and a way of viewing the fundamental problems in a discipline. Research traditions include a range of methodologies used to investigate the problems posed by the research tradition. In contrast to logical empiricism, theories and research traditions are neither solely accepted because they are empirically confirmed nor solely rejected because they are empirically disproved. Changes and debates in scientific theories often develop in the context of historical and conceptual changes such as the influence of feminism or the exposure of oppression. The concept of research traditions provides insight into the impact of the different psychosocial theories of depression and the effect of marginalization on the use of psychosocial theories of depression with individuals with I/DD.

It is useful in understanding Laudan's (1977, 1996) conceptions to discuss the contrast with the conceptions of scientific development of Kuhn (1962), whose writings provoked debates regarding the merits of logical empiricism versus historicism. According to Kuhn, scientific progress can be seen as epochs, the boundaries of which are scientific revolutions. In scientific epochs, a paradigm is supreme. Similar to Laudan, Kuhn does not see scientific progress as the methodological falsification of theories and the empirical development of new theories. Anomalies that do not fit with the precepts of a theory come up all the time. Even the most stubborn of the anomalies are usually solved by the normal science of the paradigm of that theory. The theory or paradigm goes into crisis when the anomalies build up and become more recognized by the profession, leading to crisis and the development of new theories and paradigms.

Laudan (1977, 1996), however, suggests that new theories generally do not develop because of a buildup of anomalies in old theories. Laudan specifically recognizes the influence of history, politics, and conceptual changes on science and discusses the centrality of debate about the conceptual foundations of theories. New theories and research traditions tend to integrate concepts and methods from older traditions, although the theory transitions are generally noncumulative and the logical and empirical content of older theories is generally not preserved as a whole. Rather than there being boundaries between scientific epochs and paradigms, the coexistence of rival theories and debate about them is the rule rather than the exception. Evaluation of competing research traditions is primarily comparative and should question whether newer research traditions are able to pose and answer a broader range of conceptual and empirical problems and should include discussion of the conceptual foundation of the research tradition (Laudan, 1996).

This chapter discusses the key groups of theories of depression in light of the concept of research traditions developed by Laudan (1977, 1996). Laudan (1977) identifies "Freudianism" and "behaviorism" as examples of research traditions (p. 78).

The research traditions in depression affect the practice of scientists and practitioners. In turn the practices of scientists and practitioners influence theory. The four main groups of psychosocial theories of depression reflect different conceptions of human nature, developed in different eras, reflect the historical and conceptual changes of those eras, and continue to coexist. The development and use of theories in the various research traditions with individuals with I/DD reflect their marginalization in society and are intertwined with questions of the history of care of individuals with I/DD and the thinking and practices of science in historical eras.

RESEARCH TRADITIONS OF PSYCHOSOCIAL THEORIES OF DEPRESSION

Psychodynamic/Psychoanalytic Theories of Depression and Intellectual Disability

Psychodynamic/psychoanalytic theories are based on the writings of Freud (1917/1986) and Abraham (1911/1986). Core concepts include the existence of unconscious processes and motivation. This group of theories views behaviors as based on early development and as often unconscious (Clark et al., 1999). Anger or hostility (retroflected anger) turned inward and connected to unconsciously identified object loss is related to depression (Dowd, 2002). Psychodynamic/psychoanalytic theories place emphasis on ego deficiencies and the lack of loving relationships with the mother in the development of depression (Clark et al.). Therapies are often directed at uncovering and resolving unconscious processes and early childhood experiences.

The development of psychodynamic/psychoanalytic theories was revolutionary at the time. Prior to this, it was assumed that humans always understood their behaviors and that children were little adults (Dowd, 2002). Psychodynamic/psychoanalytic theories and treatments were dominant in psychopathology research and treatment in the general population until the 1960s. For individuals with I/DD, psychodynamic theories of depression were used, although not widely (Chidester & Menninger, 1936). Research with psychodynamic/psychoanalytic theories consisted largely of anecdotal reports and case studies (Levitas & Gilson, 1989).

Psychodynamic/psychoanalytic theories led to the development of related therapies. The therapies are protracted and bias existed dismissing the possibility of psychodynamic/psychoanalytic therapies in individuals with I/DD because of the impairments in communication and lack of self-reliance (Rogers & Dymond, 1954). Starting in the 1950s, the limited use of psychodynamic/psychoanalytic theories and techniques was largely dropped with individuals with I/DD (Paniagua & DeFazio, 1989).

The psychodynamic/psychoanalytic view of human nature includes the overemphasis on unconscious processes and suppressed early childhood experiences on depression and the neglect of the effect of conscious cognitive processes, social learning, life experiences, and neurobiology (Clark et al., 1999). As with the general population, these are important factors in depression for individuals with I/DD.

Behavioral Theories of Depression and Intellectual Disability

Behavior modification, especially operant conditioning, became the dominant mode of treatment of psychopathology for individuals with I/DD during the 1950s (Matson & Coe, 1992). Behavioral conceptions and theories of depression and other psychopathology focus on observable behavior in relation to the environmental stimuli shaping the behaviors, specifically the antecedents and consequences of behavior (Clark et al., 1999). Depression is thought to be an overgeneralized response to a loss or reduction of positive reinforcement in the environment. Skinner (1978), an early behavioral theorist, specifically argued that he was not interested in the effects of conscious cognition but solely in behavior and how environment influences behavior.

Laudan (1977, 1996) argued that history and practices in historical eras often have influence on the development of research traditions. The widespread use of behavioral theories and treatments with individuals with I/DD in the 1950s had more to do with history than with the disproving of earlier psychodynamic/psychoanalytic theories and therapies. Behavior modification strategies emerged at a time of great need (Matson & Coe, 1992). Institutionalization was the norm and institutions were large, overcrowded, and understaffed. By the 1950s, operant conditioning strategies were available and shown to have some success in other areas such as toilet training and self-feeding (Matson & Coe, 1992). Behavioral therapies do not necessarily require the conscious participation of the client, and individuals with I/DD were thought to be unable to communicate and participate in their own treatment. Further psychodynamic/psychoanalytic therapies are time-consuming while behavioral therapies are relatively brief. The successes of behavior modification along with advances in pharmacology in the 1950s made it possible to treat large numbers of people with I/DD (Matson & Coe). The concentration of large numbers of people in institutions also made treatment more important for their management.

Three major behavioral theories used with individuals with I/DD include operant conditioning (Skinner, 1978), Lewinsohn's (1974) behavioral theory of depression which focused on social skills, and Seligman and associates' (Overmier & Seligman, 1967; Seligman & Maier, 1967) learned helplessness theory of depression.

Operant Conditioning. Skinner's (1978) functional model of operant conditioning was and remains a major influence in the research and treatment of individuals with I/DD (Matson & Coe, 1992). Operant conditioning strategies such as verbal and physical prompts, modeling, and token economies are well established in various aspects of the lives of individuals with I/DD, including mental health care. Skinner's principles of operant conditioning include analyzing behaviors in the context of settings, analyzing the antecedents and consequences of behaviors, and the implementation of positive and negative reinforcement to develop desired behaviors (Matson & Coe). Skinner conducted both animal and human studies, and some of the earliest human experiments were with individuals with I/DD. The principles have been used in research and treatment of depression with individuals with I/DD. Based on behavioral conceptions of depression, Matson (1982), in a classic study, identified behaviors associated with depression and rewarded non-depressed behaviors with token economies. In this study, behavior modification was effective and its effects were maintained for up to 6 months with four adults with I/DD and depression who had not responded to antidepressant medication (Matson). Matson and Coe (1992) note that the field of intellectual disabilities has seen "the most complete realization of Skinnerian psychology" (p. 185).

Lewinsohn's Behavioral Theory of Depression. Lewinsohn's (1974) behavioral theory of depression focused on the role of social skills in depression, and this theory also influenced research and discussion about depression in individuals with I/DD. In early conceptions of the theory, depression is brought on by a low rate of positive reinforcement or a high rate of aversive experiences (Lewinsohn, 1974). Positive reinforcement is a function of events that are reinforcing for the individual, the availability of reinforcement, and the social skills of the individual necessary to elicit reinforcement. It was hypothesized that depressed persons have lower social skills and less social reinforcement than nondepressed persons (Libet & Lewinsohn, 1973). Early forms of social skills training focused on specific and learned behaviors in specific situations (McFall, 1982).

Based on Lewinsohn's (1974) behavioral theory of depression, Helsel and Matson (1988) theorized that the rate of depression among individuals with I/DD was likely to be greater than the rate among the general population. Further, with individuals with I/DD, research has consistently demonstrated an association between depression and difficulties with social skills (Helsel & Matson, 1988; Matson et al., 1998). Little research exists, however, on the application of social skills training to treatment of depression using behavioral models among individuals with I/DD.

Learned Helplessness Theory of Depression and Intellectual Disability. The theory of learned helplessness was an influential behavioral theory of depression and affected thinking about depression and individuals with I/DD. The term "learned helplessness" was first used to describe the debilitated escape-avoidance response shown by dogs exposed to uncontrollable shocks in the laboratory (Overmier & Seligman, 1967; Seligman & Maier, 1967). Animals unable to control negative stimuli developed behaviors consistent with depression. Seligman and associates argued that learned helplessness plays a part in a wide variety of human conditions, including depression. The theory generated an enormous amount of research in the general population (Ingram, Miranda, & Segal, 1998).

Early research on depression with individuals with I/DD also proposed that learned helplessness is relevant to understanding their experience. Reynolds and Miller (1985) found that a group of adolescents with mild I/DD scored higher on both depressive symptoms and learned helplessness than a matched group of adolescents without I/DD. Individuals with I/DD exhibit more helplessness than their nondisabled peers (Gargiulo & O'Sullivan, 1986). No research was found on treatment interventions for depression for individuals with I/DD based on this theory. Both social skills theory of depression and learned helplessness theory of depression were later reconceptualized as cognitive theories of depression (Clark et al., 1999).

Critique of behavioral theories of depression. Behavioral theories of depression continue to be a major influence in the treatment of depression and other mental health disorders for individuals with I/DD (Dosen & Day, 2001), but many problems exist with behavioral theories and treatment strategies. A general issue is the view of behavioral theories of depression of human nature, particularly the environmental determinism and the denial of cognitive processes in depression, and in behavior in general. As well, a major theme of behavior modification literature is punishment strategies in which there are significant ethical and legal concerns, and most studies of behavior modification have been conducted in controlled environments where effectiveness, maintenance, and generalizations to new environments are problematic (Nezu & Nezu, 1994).

Cognitive Theories of Depression and Intellectual Disability

In the late 1960s and 1970s, especially in the United States, there was a reaction against the narrow conceptualizations of behaviorism (Dowd, 2002), and there was also controversy regarding the effectiveness of psychodynamic/psychoanalytic therapies (Clark et al., 1999; Dowd, 2002). Important changes in clinical theory and practice in the era paved the way for the development of cognitive theories of depression. One was the development of social learning theory by Bandura (1977a, 1977b; see also Clark et al.; Dowd). Another was the development of cognitive psychotherapies by both psychoanalytically trained clinicians and researchers and behaviorally trained clinicians and researchers (Clark et al.; Dowd). Beck and Ellis were both psychoanalytically trained and independently developed cognitive therapies of depression (Beck, 1967) and rational-emotive therapy (Ellis, 1962). Behaviorally trained clinicians and researchers developed cognitive-behavioral interventions such as problem-solving therapy (D'Zurilla & Goldfried, 1971) and stress-inoculation training (Meichenbaum, 1977). This work brought an emphasis to the interaction of the person and cognitive interpretations of the environment and on cognitive processes in the development of depression (Clark et al.; Dowd).

In contrast to psychodynamic/psychotherapeutic and behavioral theories, cognitive theories of depression emphasize the role of conscious thought processes and social learning on depression. A basic assumption of cognitive theories is that humans respond primarily to cognitive interpretations of the environment rather than to the environment itself. Human construction of meaning influences all emotional and behavioral experience (Beck, Rush, Shaw, & Emery, 1979; Clark et al., 1999).

Cognitive theory and cognitive therapies do integrate aspects of earlier psychodynamic/psychotherapeutic and behavioral theories such as the significance of early childhood experience, hostility and anger turned inward, and the role of social reinforcement (Clark et al., 1999). Cognitive therapy differs from psychodynamic/psychoanalytic therapy, however, in its emphasis on here-and-now problems. It does not dwell on unconscious factors or childhood recollections (Beck et al., 1979). While behavior modification techniques are also usually a part of cognitive therapy, cognitive therapy differs from behavior therapy in its emphasis on internal experiences, such as thoughts, feelings, and attitudes (Beck et al.).

Depression is seen as a consequence of negative thoughts (Clark et al., 1999). In cognitive theories, there is a cognitive triad: an individual's negative view of himself/herself, the interpretation of experiences in a negative way, and a negative view of the future (Clark et al.). In cognitive therapy, emphasis is put on changing or modifying the client's internal experiences, thoughts, feelings, and attitudes (Clark et al.). The explication of cognitive theory has led to extensive development of research and treatment in the general population over the last 30 years (Ingram et al., 1998).

Reformulation of Social Skills and Learned Helplessness Theories. Laudan (1984) discusses that changes from one research tradition to another often involve changes in the views of scientists regarding the nature of reality, in the value systems of scientists and in their methodologies. Potential avenues of change include modification of some of the theories in a research tradition and changes in core views of the research tradition (Laudan, 1977). In light of the criticisms of value systems and views of reality of behavioral theories, it is of note that both Lewinsohn's behavioral theory of depression focusing on social skills and Seligman and associates' learned helplessness theory of depression were reformulated as cognitive theories (Clark et al., 1999). For example, McFall (1982) wrote a classic article critiquing molecular behavioral models of social skills theory and proposed information processing models. A central role was proposed for social learning in mediation of interpersonal social skill difficulties and treatment of depression (Lewinsohn, Antonuccio, Breckenridge, & Teri, 1984).

Learned Helplessness Theory was Reformulated as a Cognitive Theory of Depression. Abramson and associates proposed that exposure to uncontrollable events alone is insufficient to produce the deficits associated with helplessness, and that cognitive concepts account for individual differences in response to uncontrollability (Abramson, Alloy, & Metalsky, 1988). Attributional style is hypothesized as a key causal factor in depression, and the phenomenon of learned helplessness is shown only if an individual generalizes the expectation to a new controllable situation (Abramson, Seligman, & Teasdale, 1978). According to the reformulated learned helplessness theory, how stable and global depressed individuals perceive their helplessness is associated with how general and chronic the depression is (Abramson et al., 1978). Learned helplessness theory has been further reformulated as hopelessness theory of depression, a diasthesis-stress model of depression (Abramson, Metalsky, & Alloy, 1989), and its authors identify it as one of the two major cognitive etiological theories of depression (Abramson et al., 1988).

Implications of Cognitive Theories of Depression. While cognitive theories have been used in research and treatment of depression since the late 1960s, the use of these theories with individuals with I/DD developed later. In conjunction with the general acceptance that individuals with I/DD have depressive disorders, research using cognitive theories of depression with individuals with I/DD developed since the mid-1980s. The research has established that cognition is also involved in depression in individuals with mild and moderate I/DD. For example, in individuals with I/DD, depression is associated with negative self-concept (Benson & Ivins, 1992), frequency of automatic negative thoughts, thoughts of hopelessness, and self-reinforcement (Nezu, Nezu, Rotherburg, DelliCarpini, & Groag, 1995), social comparison (Dagnan & Sandhu, 1999), and self-hatred (Ailey, 2002). Conversely, the absence of depression in adolescents with I/DD is associated with global self-worth and positive self-image (Zigler, Bennet-Gates, & Hodapp, 1999).

Cognitive therapies are increasingly used for individuals with mild and moderate I/DD (Benson & Valenti-Hein, 2001; Nezu et al., 1995). The cognitive-behavioral therapies of self-instruction, problem-solving, modeling, and relaxation training have all been used with success for mental health disorders with individuals with I/DD (Benson & Valenti-Hein, 2001). As well, research regarding social skills and problem solving training demonstrates that using cognitive interventions improves social interactions and social problem-solving for individuals with I/DD (Castles & Glass, 1986), although research on the efficacy or mechanisms of social skills training programs using cognitive interventions in the treatment of depression was not found. Nevertheless, the cognitive theories of depression do not deal well with the social experiences of individuals with I/DD and the relationship of those experiences to depression.

Critique of Cognitive Theories of Depression. Over the last 25 years, significant theoretical work in depression and other fields raises conceptual concerns with cognitive theories of depression. Bowlby's (1969, 1980) work hypothesizing a universal psychobiologically based need for relatedness brought a focus of attention to the social experiences and consequences of depression (Hammen, 1999). The work of Bowlby also looked at issues in childhood in a different way than psychodynamic/psychoanalytic theories and promoted interest in the childhood origins of vulnerability to depression related to problems in attachment (Hammen). Brown and Harris' (1978) "Social Origins of Depression" examined women's experience associated with an increased risk of depression. Before the work of Brown and Harris, life stress research proceeded in relative isolation from cognitive models of depression (Hammen). The works of Bowlby and Brown and Harris stimulated discussion of conceptual problems with cognitive theories of depression, the most general problem being the overfocus on internal cognitive processes and intrapersonal factors in depression and the lack of focus on interpersonal and social factors (Hammen).

Interpersonal/Ecological Theories of Depression

Interpersonal/ecological theories of depression are based on conceptual and empirical work highlighting the importance of relationships and the social risk factors of depression, as well as critiques of cognitive theories of depression (Hammen, 1999). In interpersonal theories, social relationships and their context and social and environmental conditions are viewed as critical features of vulnerability to depression. Interpersonal theories view a need for relationships as integral to human nature, and address the context of relationships that may be particular to groups, as well as how the context may affect depression (Hammen).

Within the research tradition of interpersonal/ecological theories of depression there are various theories and models. These include the sociophysiological perspective of Gardner and Price (1999), a theory of self-silencing and women's depression (Jack, 1999), and a model of depression based on the Theory of Human Relatedness (Hagerty, Lynch-Sauer, Patusky, & Bouwsema, 1993; Hagerty & Williams, 1999). A common feature of these theories and models is that interpersonal factors are part of the development of depression (Joiner et al., 1999).

Interpersonal Critique of Social Skills and Learned Helplessness Theories of Depression. In light of the critique of cognitive theories of depression, it is of note that the role of social skills in depression and learned helplessness/hopelessness theory are currently being reevaluated in the context of interpersonal theories of depression (Ingram et al., 1998; Trower, 1995). Trower critiques the information processing models of social skills as not containing an interpersonal theory within them, criticizes the asocial emphasis in social skills assessment of decontextualized "sick" and "malfunctioning" individuals, and calls for a paradigm shift in social skills theory.

The work of Coyne (1999) and Coyne and Calarco (1995) regarding social skills and depression should be noted in the context of the reevaluation of social skills theory. In the general population, Coyne and Calarco found support for the hypothesis that the experience of depression affects the evaluation of individuals with depression about their prospects of social relationships and that such evaluations cause them to place limits on their social relationships. The limits placed on social relationships may increase the immediate vulnerability to recurrence of depression (Coyne & Calarco). Loss events that provoke depression may also deplete social resources and contribute to skills deficits. Further, as a result of the effects of the individuals with depression on others, individuals with depression may face environments in which they have to exert more effort to maintain social relationships (Coyne). Thus, the social performance deficits of individuals with depression should not automatically be interpreted as social skills deficits but as a complex interaction of the individuals with depression and their environment (Coyne). The analysis of the social skills deficits of individuals with I/DD should also include an analysis of the context of the deficits (Sherman, Sheldon, Harchik, Edwards, & Quinn, 1992).

Cognitive models of learned helplessness/hopelessness theory are also currently critiqued in light of interpersonal/ecological theories of depression. In a classic article, Coyne and Gotlib (1983) reviewed research on the role of cognitive functions in depression and specifically learned helplessness theory, and found problems with empirical validation of the theory. Differences in ratings of control and in performance expectations between depressed and nondepressed persons were not as great as hypothesized (Coyne & Gotlib, 1983). Ingram and colleagues (1998) reviewed research and found that learned helplessness/hopelessness theory fails to demonstrate clearly that attributional style is present prior to an episode of depression. Learned helplessness may develop along with depression as part of the interpersonal effects of depression.

The reevaluation of the role of social skills and learned helplessness/hopelessness theory indicates the potential benefit of using interpersonal/ecological theories of depression. Interpersonal/ecological theories may help to reevaluate research on social skills deficits and learned helplessness in the light of social conditions in which individuals with I/DD have decreased opportunities to develop social skills and have an increased experience of and expectation of failure. Increased risk of depression and social skills deficits may both be related to environmental and social conditions.

Interpersonal/Ecological Theories of Depression and Individuals With I/DD. Interpersonal/ecological theories of depression are only now beginning to be used with individuals with I/DD (Ailey, 2002), reflecting the continued marginalization of this group of individuals. However, over the last 20 years, research demonstrates that major interpersonal concepts are important in depression for individuals with I/DD. Individuals with I/DD are aware of social stigma (Reiss & Benson, 1984) and often face loneliness and limited social networks (Krauss, Seltzer, & Goodman, 1992). Negative social support and social strain are associated with mental health disorders in individuals with I/DD (Lunsky & Havercamp, 1999; Nezu et al., 1995). Loneliness and life satisfaction are associated with depression in individuals with Down syndrome (Ailey). Interpersonal/ecological theories may help to integrate current knowledge regarding cognitive vulnerability to depression with individuals with I/DD with a focus on the interpersonal context of their lives.

Other indications support the important role of interpersonal/ecological theories in developing research and treatment of depression with individuals with I/DD. In interpersonal theories of depression, social and environmental factors are risk factors for mental health disorders and include major life changes, isolation, stigmatization, history of abuse, and social and family stress. Research indicates that social and environmental risk factors play a role in depression for individuals with I/DD. For example, Hollins and Esterhuyzen (1997) found that 26% of a group of individuals with I/DD who had lost a parent within 2 years could be characterized as depressed. Heyman, Swain, Gilman, Handyside, and Neyman (1997) conducted a qualitative study among adults with mental retardation. The study assessed some of the context in which these adults had what was labeled as "challenging" and "problematic" behavior. The authors noted that the "problematic" behavior was often the result of trying to maintain nonconfirmed identities and self-worth in adverse circumstances.

CONCLUSION

The historicist worldview indicates the need to assess the impact of marginalization on nursing theory and practice. The concept of marginalization assists the discipline of nursing in understanding the complexities of vulnerability and health (Hall et al., 1994). Individuals with I/DD continue to be marginalized in American society, and the way in which theories and treatment models of depression are used with this population contributes to the persistence of marginalization. Despite improvements in the recognition of the need for mental health care for individuals with I/DD, behaviors continue to be the primary reason for entry into the mental health system, individuals with I/DD continue to face inappropriate medication use for chemical restraint of behaviors, and mental health disorders not manifested by problematic behaviors may not be treated.

Research traditions strongly influence the empirical and conceptual problems posed by theories in that tradition (Laudan, 1977). In mental health care, behavioral and cognitive research traditions are limited in terms of providing insight into the empirical and conceptual problems of the psychosocial aspects of depression and the models of treatment for individuals with I/DD. Behavioral theories fail to take account of the complex relationship of the individual with the environment or the role of the conscious interaction of the individual with the environment. The increased focus on cognitive manifestations of depression in individuals with I/DD has broadened the focus of mental health care but does not take adequate account of the impact of social conditions on the mental health of this population.

Interpersonal/ecological theories of depression pose a broader range of conceptual and empirical problems that are important to individuals with I/DD as they explicitly recognize a universal basic human need for relatedness. With the focus on social conditions and human needs for relatedness, interpersonal/ecological theories of depression may assist in ending an overfocus on behaviors in mental health treatment for individuals with intellectual disabilities and provide better means of assessing the relationship of behaviors to the environment and overall mental health. Further, interpersonal/ecological theories may provide information on reasons for the increased risk of depression among individuals with I/DD, and help to integrate increasing knowledge regarding the cognitive manifestations of depression in individuals with I/DD with assessment of their life experiences. Interpersonal/ecological theories have the potential to broaden the focus of mental health care for depression for this population and to provide improved access to quality mental health care.

REFERENCES

Abraham, K. (1986). Notes on the psycho-analytical investigation and the treatment of manic-depressive insanity and allied conditions. Reprinted in J. C. Coyne (Ed.), *Essential papers on depression* (pp. 31-47). New York: New York University Press. (Original work published 1911)

Abramson, L. Y., Alloy, L. B., & Metalsky, G. I. (1988). The cognitive diathesis-stress theories of depression: Toward an adequate evaluation of the theories' validities. In L. B. Alloy (Ed.), *Cognitive processes in depression* (pp. 3-30). New York: The Guilford Press.

Abramson, L. Y., Metalsky, G. I., & Alloy, L. B. (1989). Hopelessness depression: A theory-based subtype of depression. *Psychological Review, 96*, 358-372.

Abramson, L. Y., Seligman, M. E. P., & Teasdale, J. D. (1978). Learned helplessness in humans: Critique and reformulation. *Journal of Abnormal Psychology, 87*, 49-74.

Ailey, S. H. (2002). *Evaluating an interpersonal model of depression in adults with Down syndrome*. Unpublished doctoral dissertation, University of Illinois at Chicago.

American Psychiatric Association. (2000). *Diagnostic and statistical manual of mental disorders* (Rev. ed.). Washington, DC: Author.

Bandura, A. (1977a). Self-efficacy: Toward a unifying theory of behavior change. *Psychological Review, 84*, 191-215.

Bandura, A. (1977b). *Social learning theory*. Englewood Cliffs, NJ: Prentice-Hall.

Beck, A. T. (1967). *Depression: Clinical, experimental and theoretical aspects.* New York: Harper & Row.

Beck, A. T., Rush, A. J., Shaw, B. F., & Emery, G. (1979). *Cognitive therapy of depression*. New York: Guilford.

Benson, B. A., & Ivins, J. (1992) Anger, depression and self-concept in adults with mental retardation. *Journal of Intellectual Disability Research, 36*, 169-175.

Benson, B. A., & Valenti-Hein, D. (2001). Cognitive and social learning treatment. In A. Dosen & K. Day (Eds.), *Treating mental illness and behavior disorders in children and adults with mental retardation* (pp.101-188). Northumberland, UK: Northgate & Prudhoe NHS Trust.

Borthwick-Duffy, S. A. (1994). Epidemiology and prevalence of psychopathology in people with mental retardation. *Journal of Consulting and Clinical Psychology, 62*, 17-27.

Bowlby, J. (1969). *Attachment and loss: Vol I: Attachment.* New York: Basic Books.

Bowlby, J. (1980). *Attachment and loss: Vol III: Loss: Sadness and depression.* London: Hogarth Press.

Brown, G. W., & Harris, T. (1978). *Social origins of depression: Study of psychiatric disorder in women*. New York: Free Press.

Castles, E. E., & Glass, C. R. (1986). Training in social and interpersonal problem-solving skills for mildly and moderately retarded adults. *American Journal of Mental Deficiency, 91*, 35-42.

Center for Disease Control. (1996). State-specific rates of mental retardation—United States, 1993. *Morbidity and Mortality Weekly Report, 45*, 61-65.

Chidester, L., & Meninger, K. (1936). The application of psychoanalytic methods to the study of mental retardation. *American Journal of Orthopsychiatry, 6*, 616-624.

Clark, D. A., Beck, A. T., & Alford, B. A. (1999). *Scientific foundations of cognitive theory and theory of depression*. New York: John Wiley & Sons.

Coyne, J. C. (1999). Thinking interactionally about depression: A radical restatement. In T. Joiner & J. C. Coyne (Eds.), *The interactional nature of depression* (pp. 365-392). Washington, DC: American Psychological Association.

Coyne, J. C., & Calarco, M. M. (1995). Effects of the experience of depression: Application of focus group and survey methodologies. *Psychiatry, 58*, 149-163.

Coyne, J. C., & Gotlib, I. H. (1983). The role of cognition in depression: A critical appraisal. *Psychological Bulletin, 94*, 472-505.

Dagnan, D., & Sandhu, S. (1999). Social comparison, self-esteem and depression in people with intellectual disability. *Journal of Intellectual Disability Research, 43*, 372-379.

Deb, S. T. M., & Bright, C. (2001). Mental disorder in adults with intellectual disability. 2: The rate of behavior disorders among a community-based population aged between 16 and 64 years. *Journal of Intellectual Disability Research, 45*, 506-514.

Dosen, A., & Day, K. (2001). Treatment: An integrative approach. In A. Dosen & K. Day (Eds.), *Treating mental illness and behavior disorders in children and adults with mental retardation* (pp. 519-528). Northumberland, UK: Northgate & Prudhoe NHS Trust.

Dowd, E. T. (2002). History and recent developments in cognitive psychotherapy. In R. L. Leahy & E. T. Dowd (Eds.), *Clinical advances in cognitive psychotherapy: Theory and application* (pp. 15-28). New York: Springer Publishing.

D'Zurilla, T. J., & Goldfried, M. R. (1971). Problem solving and behavior modification. *Journal of Abnormal Psychology, 78*, 107-126.

Edelstein, T. M., & Glenwick, D. S. (2001). Direct-care workers' attributions of psychopathology in adults with mental retardation. *Mental Retardation, 39*, 368-378.

Edwards, S. E. (1999). The idea of nursing science. *Journal of Advanced Nursing, 29*, 563-569.

Einfeld, S. I., & Aman, M. (1995). Issues in the taxonomy of psychopathology in mental retardation. *Journal of Autism and Developmental Disorder, 25*, 143-167.

Ellis, A. (1962). *Reason and emotion in psychotherapy.* New York: Lyle-Stuart.

Forbes, D. A., King, K. M., Kushner, K. E., Letourneau, N. L., Myrick, A. F., & Profetto-McGrath, J. (1999). Warrantable evidence in nursing science. *Journal of Advanced Nursing, 29*, 373-379.

Freud, S. (1986). Mourning and melancholia. In J. C. Coyne (Ed.), *Essential papers on depression* (pp. 48-63). New York: New York University Press. (Original work published 1917)

Gardner, W. I. (1967). Occurrence of severe depressive reactions in the mentally retarded. *American Journal of Psychiatry, 124*, 386-388.

Gardner, R., & Price, J. S. (1999). Sociophysiology and depression. In T. Joiner & J. C. Coyne (Eds.), *The interactional nature of depression* (pp. 247-268). Washington, DC: American Psychological Association.

Gargiulo, R. M., & O'Sullivan, P. S. (1986). Mildly mentally retarded and nonretarded children's learned helplessness. *American Journal of Mental Deficiency, 91*, 203-206.

Hagerty, B. M. K., Lynch-Sauer, J., Patusky, K. L., & Bouwsema, M. (1993). An emerging theory of human relatedness. *Image, 25*, 291-296.

Hagerty, B. M., & Williams, R. A. (1999). The effects of sense of belonging, social support, conflict, and loneliness on depression. *Nursing Research, 48*, 215-219.

Hall, J. M., Stevens, P. E., & Meleis, A. I. (1994). Marginalization: A guiding concept for valuing diversity in nursing knowledge development. *Advances in Nursing Science, 16*(4), 23-41.

Hammen, C. (1999). The emergence of an interpersonal approach to depression. In T. Joiner & J. C. Coyne (Eds.), *The interactional nature of depression* (pp. 21-36). Washington, DC: American Psychological Association.

Helsel, W. J., & Matson, J. L. (1988). The relationship of depression to social skills and intellectual functioning in mentally retarded adults. *Journal of Mental Deficiency Research, 32*, 411-418.

Heyman, B., Swain, J., Gilman, M., Handyside, E. C., & Neyman, W. (1997). Alone in the crowd: How adults with learning difficulties cope with social network problems. *Social Science in Medicine, 44*, 41-53.

Hollins, S., & Esterhuyzen, A. (1997). Bereavement and grief in adults with learning disabilities. *British Journal of Psychiatry, 170*, 497-501.

Hurley, A. D., Folstein, M., & Lam, N. (2003). Patients with and without intellectual disability seeking outpatient psychiatric services: Diagnoses and prescribing pattern. *Journal of Intellectual Disability Research, 47*, 39-50.

Ingram, R. E., Miranda, J., & Segal, Z. V. (1998). *Cognitive vulnerability to depression*. New York: Guilford Press.

Jack, D. C. (1999). Silencing the self: Inner dialogues and outer realities. In T. Joiner & J. C. Coyne (Eds.), *The interactional nature of depression* (pp. 221-246). Washington, DC: American Psychological Association.

Jelliffe, S. E. (1931). Some historical phases of the manic-depressive synthesis. *The Journal of Nervous and Mental Disease, 73*, 353-374, 499-521.

Joiner, T. E., Coyne, J. C., & Blalock, J. (1999). On the interpersonal nature of depression: Overview and synthesis. In T. Joiner & J. C. Coyne (Eds.), *The interactional nature of depression* (pp. 3-20). Washington, DC: American Psychological Association.

Kessler, R. C., Berglund, P., Demler, O., Jin, R., Koretz., D., Merikangas, K. R., et al. (2003). The epidemiology of major depressive disorder: Results from the National Comorbidity Survey Replication (NCS-R). *The Journal of the American Medical Association, 289*, 3095-3105.

Kuhn, T. S. (1962). *The structure of scientific revolutions.* Chicago: The University of Chicago Press.

Krauss, M., Seltzer, M. M., & Goodman, S. J. (1992). Social support networks of adults with mental retardation who live at home. *American Journal of Mental Retardation, 96*, 432- 441.

Laudan, L. (1977). *Progress and its problems: Towards a theory of scientific growth*. Berkeley: University of California Press.

Laudan, L. (1984). *Science and values*. Berkeley: University of California Press.

Laudan, L. (1996). *Beyond positivism and relativism*. Boulder, CO: Westview Press.

Levitas, A., & Gilson, S. (1989). Psychodynamic psychotherapy with mildly and moderately retarded persons. In R. J. Fletcher & F. J. Menolascino (Eds.), *Mental retardation and mental illness* (pp. 71-110). Lanham, MD: Lexington Books.

Lewinsohn, P. M. (1974). A behavioural approach to depression. In R. J. Friedman & M. M. Katz (Eds.), *The psychology of depression: Contemporary theory and research* (pp. 157-178). Washington, DC: Wiley.

Lewinsohn, P. M., Antonuccio, D. O., Breckenridge, J. S., & Teri, L. (1984). *The coping-with-depression course*. Eugene, OR: Castalia Publishing.

Libet, J. M., & Lewinsohn, P. M. (1973). Concept of social skill with specific reference to the behavior of depressed persons. *Journal of Consulting and Clinical Psychology, 40*, 304-312.

Lunsky, Y., & Havercamp, S. M. (1999). Distinguishing low levels of social support and social strain: Implications for dual diagnosis. *American Journal on Mental Retardation, 104*, 200-204.

Matson, J. L. (1982). The treatment of behavioral characteristics of depression in the mentally retarded. *Behavior Therapy, 13*, 209-218.

Matson, J. L., Bamburg, J. W., Matville, E. A., Pinkston, J., Bielecki, J., Kuhn, D, et al. (2000). Psychopharmacology and mental retardation: A 10 year review (1990-1999). *Research in Developmental Disabilities, 21*, 263-296.

Matson, J. L., & Coe, D. A. (1992). Applied behavior analysis: Its impact on the treatment of mentally retarded emotionally disturbed people. *Research in Developmental Disabilities, 13*, 171-189.

Matson, J. L., Smiroldo, B. B., Brandi, B., & Bamburg, J. W. (1998). The relationship of social skills to psychopathology for individuals with severe or profound mental retardation. *Journal of Intellectual and Developmental Disabilities, 23*, 137-145.

McFall, R. M. (1982). A review and reformation of the concept of social skills. *Behavioral Assessment, 4*, 1-33.

Meichenbaum, D. B. (1977). *Cognitive-behavior modification: An integrative approach.* New York: Plenum Press.

Meins, W. (1993). Prevalence and risk factors for depressive disorders in adults with intellectual disability. *Australia and New Zealand Journal of Developmental Disabilities, 18*, 147-156.

Nezu, C. M., & Nezu, A. M. (1994). Outpatient psychotherapy for adults with mental retardation and concomitant psychopathology: Research and clinical imperatives. *Journal of Consulting and Clinical Psychology, 62*, 34-42.

Nezu, C. M., Nezu, A. M., Rotherburg, J. L., DelliCarpini, L., & Groag, I. (1995). Depression in adults with mild mental retardation: Are cognitive variables involved? *Cognitive Therapy and Research, 19*, 227-239.

Overmier, J. B., & Seligman, M. E. (1967). Effects of inescapable shock upon subsequent escape and avoidance responding. *Journal of Comparative and Physiological Psychology, 63*, 28-33.

Paniagua, C., & De Fazio, A. (1989). Psychodynamics of the mildly mentally retarded and borderline-intelligence adult. In R. J. Fletcher & F. J. Menolascino (Eds.), *Mental retardation and mental illness* (pp. 35-58). Lanham, MD: Lexington Books.

Papineau, D. (1996). *The philosophy of science*. New York: Oxford University Press.

Reed, P. G. (1995). A treatise on nursing knowledge development for the 21st century: Beyond postmodernism. *Advances in Nursing Science, 17*(3), 70-84.

Reiss, S., & Benson, B. A. (1984). Awareness of negative social conditions among mentally retarded, emotionally disturbed outpatients. *American Journal of Psychiatry, 141*, 88-90.

Reiss, S., & Rojahn, J. (1993). Joint occurrence of depression and aggression in children and adults with mental retardation. *Journal of Intellectual Disability Research, 37*, 287-294.

Reynolds, W. M., & Miller, K. L. (1985). Depression and learned helplessness in mentally retarded and nonmentally retarded adolescents: An initial investigation. *Applied Research in Mental Retardation, 6*, 295-306.

Rogers, C. R., & Dymond, R. F. (1954). *Psychotherapy and personality change.* Chicago: University of Chicago Press.

Seligman, M. E., & Maier, S. F. (1967). Failure to escape traumatic shock. *Journal of Experimental Psychology, 74*, 1-9.

Sherman, J. A., Sheldon, J. B., Harchik, A. E., Edwards, K., & Quinn, J. M. (1992). Social evaluation of behaviors comprising three social skills and a comparison of the performance of people with and without mental retardation. *American Journal on Mental Retardation, 96*, 419-441.

Silva, M. C., & Rothbart, D. (1984). An analysis of changing trends in philosophies of science on nursing theory development and testing. *Advances in Nursing Science, 6*(2),1-13.

Skinner, B. F. (1978). *Reflections on behaviorism and society*. Englewood Cliffs, NJ: Prentice-Hall.

Sovner, R., & Pary, R. J. (1993). Affective disorders in developmentally disabled persons. In J. L. Matson & R. P. Barrett (Eds.), *Psychopathology in the mentally retarded* (pp. 87-147). Needham Heights, MA: Allyn & Bacon.

Szymanski, L., & King, B. H. (1999). Practice parameters for the assessment and treatment of children, adolescents, and adults with mental retardation and comorbid mental disorders. *Journal of the American Academy of Child and Adolescent Psychiatry, 38*(Suppl. 12), 5S-31S.

Trent, J. W. (1994). *Inventing the feeble mind: A history of mental retardation in the United States*. Berkeley: University of California Press.

Trower, P. (1995). Adult social skills: State of the art and future directions. In W. O'Donohue & L. Krasner (Eds.), *Handbook of psychological skills training* (pp. 54- 80). Needham Heights, MA: Allyn & Bacon.

Whall, A. L., & Hicks, F. D. (2002). The unrecognized paradigm shift in nursing: Implications, problems, and possibilities. *Nursing Outlook, 50*, 72-76.

Zigler, E., Bennett-Gates, D., & Hodapp, R. M. (1999). Assessing personality traits of individuals with mental retardation. In E. Zigler & D. Bennett-Gates (Eds.), *Personality development in individuals with mental retardation* (pp. 206-225). New York: Cambridge University Press.

Acknowledgments. This chapter is based in part on literature review for a doctoral dissertation submitted to the Graduate College of the University of Illinois at Chicago by the first author, dissertation chair Dr. Arlene Miller. The authors acknowledge the advice and assistance of members of the dissertation committee: Dr. Tamar Heller, Dr. Julia Cowell, Dr. Everett Smith, Dr. Shu-pi Chen, and Dr. Theresa Savage. The authors would also like to thank Dr. Mary Johnson for her review and suggestions for this chapter.

3

Maternal Postpartum Depression Symptoms: A Longitudinal Study

June Andrews Horowitz
Janice Goodman

Postpartum depression and postpartum depression symptoms occur during the critical period of the first months of infants' lives, compromising maternal functioning and the developing mother-infant relationship (C. Beck, 1995, 1998; Field, 1995; Weinberg et al., 2001). Moreover, for some women depression symptoms linger beyond the early postpartum period (Beeghly et al., 2002; Josefsson, Berg, Nordin, & Sydsjo, 2001; Small, Brown, Lumley, & Astbury, 1994). However, despite the negative consequences associated with postpartum depression symptoms, only limited longitudinal data are available concerning the course of maternal depression symptoms.

The purpose of this study was to examine changes in maternal depression symptoms over time from the postpartum period (i.e., 4-8 weeks, 10-14 weeks, 14-18 weeks after delivery) to 2 years after delivery among a sample of women identified with elevated depression symptoms at 2 to 4 weeks postpartum. The research questions addressed were:

1. Did women's depression scores change significantly over time?
2. What maternal factors were associated with ongoing postpartum depression symptoms at 2 years after childbirth?

BACKGROUND AND SIGNIFICANCE

Prevalence and Course of Postpartum Depression

Postpartum depression is a devastating disorder that features depressed mood, anxiety, compulsive thoughts, difficulty concentrating, poor sleep even when the baby is sleeping, poor appetite, agitation, irritability, loss of control, feelings of inadequacy, inability to cope, irrational fears, fatigue, loss of libido, feelings of guilt, and despair (Horowitz, Damato, Solon, von Metzsch, & Gill, 1995; Miller, 2002; Sichel, 2000). Many researchers have assessed the prevalence of postpartum depression and depressive symptoms at early postpartum time points (e.g., Bagedahl-Strindlund & Monsen Borjesson, 1998; Georgiopoulos et al., 1999; Lane et al., 1997; Yonkers et al., 2001). A meta-analysis of the prevalence rates of postpartum depression has indicated that an estimated 13% of new mothers experience clinical depression during the first few months postpartum (O'Hara & Swain, 1996). The prevalence may be as high as 26% among adolescent mothers (Troutman & Cutrona, 1990), and as high as 38.2% among lower socioeconomic status first-time mothers (Hobfoll, Ritter, Lavin, Hulsizer, & Cameron, 1995). In addition, as many as 28% (Horowitz, Damato, Solon, & von Metzsch, 1996) to 50% (Affonso et al., 1992) of postpartum women have reported nonclinical levels of depressive symptoms.

Assessments made after the first few postpartum months indicate that depression may extend into the first and second years after the birth of a baby (Campbell & Cohn, 1997; Small et al., 1994). In community samples, as many as 9.1% to 38.2% of women experienced depressive symptoms at 6 months postpartum (Brown & Lumley, 2000; Evans, Heron, Francomb, Oke, & Golding, 2001; Seguin, Potvin, St.-Denis, & Loiselle, 1999). In clinical samples, 30% to 54% of women who were depressed at earlier postpartum assessments were still depressed 6 months after delivery (Beeghly et al., 2002; Campbell & Cohn, 1997; Whiffen & Gotlib, 1993; Zelkowitz & Milet, 2001). Josefsson and colleagues (2001) found that among a sample of 1,558 women in Sweden, 13% had scores in the depressive range as measured by the EPDS at 6 to 8 weeks postpartum, and the percentage of women experiencing elevated depression symptoms did not decrease during the first 6 months postpartum.

Prevalence estimates of postpartum depression between 6 and 12 months postpartum have ranged from 8.1% (Evans et al., 2001) to 15.4% (Small et al., 1994). An even higher percentage of women has reported subclinical levels of depression during the second half of the first postpartum year (Hiscock & Wake, 2001). When McIntosh (1993) used a broad definition of depression (i.e., experience of depressed mood for at least 14 days after the first postpartum week), he found that 63% of women studied experienced depression at some time during the 9 months following delivery. Moreover, depressive experiences were not transient: 69% lasted more than 3 months and 47% continued for 7 or more months. Matthey, Barnett, Ungerer, and Waters (2000) reported a point prevalence of 12.4% for maternal depression at 1 year postpartum in a community-based sample. Period prevalence estimates over the first year postpartum have ranged from 27.3% (Matthey et al.) to 49% (Areias, Kumar, Barros, & Figueredo, 1996). Thus, available findings indicate that a large percentage of women experience depressive symptoms during the first year after childbirth.

Results from a small number of studies demonstrated that for a large percentage of affected women depression levels were highest in the first few months postpartum and then decreased significantly; however, depressive symptoms that persisted after the first few months postpartum tended to remain throughout the first year, and lingered throughout the second year with little change in symptom severity. Beeghly and colleagues (2002) reported that maternal depression scores were highest at 2 months postpartum and did not change significantly from 3 to 12 months postpartum. Small and colleagues (1994) found that 34% of women who were depressed at 8 to 9 months postpartum were still depressed when their child was about 2 years old. Campbell and Cohn (1997) reported that at 18 months after delivery, 18% of the women who were depressed at 2 months postpartum still met diagnostic criteria for major depression and 31% met criteria for minor depression. At 24 months, 13% met criteria for major depression and 35% for minor depression. These findings indicate that for many women, depression symptoms persist at clinical and subclinical levels through the first and second years postpartum.

Contributing Factors

Combinations of risk factors are likely to contribute to any individual woman's vulnerability to postpartum depression (PPD). Maternal prenatal depression or anxiety, history of depression, child care stress, poor marital or partner relationship, low social support, and life stress are the most consistently identified predictors of PPD. Other factors such as socioeconomic status and infant temperament are identified less consistently and tend to have smaller effect sizes in relation to PPD (C. Beck, 1996, 2001; Nielson, Videbech, Hedegaard, Dalby, & Secher, 2000; O'Hara & Swain, 1996). Although socioeconomic status has not been a strong predictor of PPD in all studies, some researchers have found elevated PPD rates ranging from 23% (Hobfoll et al., 1995) to 38% (Seguin et al., 1999) among women with very limited economic resources. Parity and age have not been consistent predictors of PPD, but younger mothers (Troutman & Cutrona, 1990) and first-time mothers (Hobfoll et al.) may experience higher rates of PPD, suggesting that maternal age and parity may be risk factors worthy of ongoing evaluation. Ethnicity and race generally have not been significant predictors of PPD in United States studies (Yonkers et al., 2001).

Some researchers have investigated factors that influence severity or course of postpartum depression. Higher depression scores in the early postpartum period have been associated with higher scores later in the first postpartum year (Beeghly et al., 2002). Prior history of depression has not been associated with persistence of postpartum depression in some studies (Campbell & Cohn, 1997; Zelkowitz & Milet, 2001); however, onset of depressive symptoms before or during pregnancy has been related to a more chronic course of depression (Zelkowitz & Milet). Low socioeconomic status and chronic stressors, such as maternal health problems, infant difficulty, lack of money, and poor social support, also have been associated with more long-lasting postpartum depression (Seguin et al., 1999).

Effects of Maternal Depression on Family Health

Persistent clinical and subclinical depression symptoms that originated during the postpartum period have significant deleterious effects on women and their families.

Depressed mood and affect are associated with poorer adaptive functioning among postpartum women and with significant deleterious effects on the affected woman's family (Weinberg et al., 2001). Men whose partners are depressed are at significantly higher risk of becoming depressed themselves (Areias et al., 1996; Ballard, Davis, Cullen, Mohan, & Dean, 1994; Deater-Deckard, Pickering, Dunn, & Golding, 1998). Postpartum depression compromises the mother-infant relationship and children's healthy development (C. Beck, 1995, 1998; Field, 1995). Campbell, Cohn, and Meyers (1995) demonstrated that women whose depression persisted through 6 months postpartum had less positive interactions with their infants than women whose depressive symptoms remitted before 6 months. Severity and chronicity of maternal depression have been related to negative child outcomes (Brennan et al., 2000; Campbell et al.; Teti, Messinger, Gelfand, & Isabella, 1995).

Thus, results of research indicate that ongoing maternal depression extends problematic effects on mothers and families; however, longitudinal research beyond the first postpartum year is limited. Furthermore, a definitive profile of contributing factors to ongoing maternal depression is lacking, although several factors, including low income, history of depression, poor social support, and high parental stress, have been identified in the literature as potential predictors; parity and younger maternal age have been inconsistent predictors. By conducting a longitudinal examination of women's depression scores, and exploring factors related to depression severity at 2 years after delivery, knowledge may be generated about postpartum depression course during an important period for parenting and early child development.

METHOD

Design

Researchers used a longitudinal within-subjects design to examine changes in maternal depression symptoms over time, and to explore factors predictive of depression symptoms at 2 years after delivery.

Measures

Demographic Information Sheet. A Demographic Information Sheet (Horowitz et al., 2001) was used for eliciting demographic and situational information. One item elicited mothers' ratings of the adequacy of overall social support. Information elicited from items was used to describe the participants and to measure the following potential predictors of depression symptoms at 2 years postpartum; maternal age, parity, income, depression history, and overall support.

Edinburgh Postnatal Depression Scale. The Edinburgh Postnatal Depression Scale (EPDS; Cox, Holden, & Sagovsky, 1987) was used to screen postpartum women for elevated depression symptoms at 2 to 4 weeks postpartum. The EPDS was designed to identify symptoms of postpartum depression and has been used widely as a screening instrument in community-based populations (Horowitz et al., 1995). The EPDS is the most frequently used measure of postpartum depression in studies conducted around the world (Affonso, De, Horowitz, & Mayberry, 2000), has demonstrated validity and reliability, and has shown sensitivity to changes in depression over time (Cox et al., 1987). The instrument consists of 10 statements describing depressive symptoms with four possible responses, each graded according to severity or duration. It takes 5 minutes to complete. Scores on the EPDS range from 0 to 30. The authors of the EPDS have recommended using 9/10 as a cutoff score to reduce failed detection to less than 10%. They have suggested that mental health referral is indicated whenever a woman scores 13 or higher. A cutoff score of 10 or greater was selected as the inclusion criterion. Cronbach's alpha was .81 for the screening administration in this study.

Beck Depression Inventory-II. The Beck Depression Inventory-II (BDI-II; Beck, Steer, & Brown, 1996) was used to measure presence and severity of depression symptoms at 4 to 8 weeks (Time 1), 10 to 14 weeks (Time 2), 14 to 18 weeks (Time 3), and 2 years (Time 4) postpartum. The BDI is a widely validated 21-item self-report scale to measure the presence and intensity of depressive symptoms. Aaron T. Beck and colleagues (A. Beck, Steer, & Garbin, 1988; A. Beck, Ward, Mendelson, Mock, & Erbaugh, 1961) demonstrated the BDI's internal consistency, split-half reliability, instrument stability, and criterion-related validity. In addition, agreement among psychiatrists' ratings within a point on a 4-point scale in 97% of the cases demonstrated the validity of the BDI as a measure of depression severity. As the standard for self-rating depression instruments, the BDI has been used as a measure of perinatal depressive symptoms in many studies (Horowitz et al., 1995). The updated BDI-II reflects current diagnostic criteria, and reliability, validity, and scoring of the original BDI and the BDI-II are comparable (A. Beck et al., 1996). In this study, Cronbach's alphas were .89, .87, .88, and .92 for Times 1 through 4 respectively.

Parenting Stress Index—Short Form. The Parenting Stress Index—Short Form (PSI/SF; Abindin, 1995) was used to assess level of parent stress at the Time 4 data collection. The PSI/SF is a widely used, self-report, 36-item instrument developed to identify potentially dysfunctional parent-child relationships that may place a child at risk for emotional disturbance, and to measure the relative magnitude of stress in the parent-child relationship. The PSI/SF is scored on a 5-point Likert scale and takes approximately 10 minutes to complete. Abidin reported extensive efforts to demonstrate validity and reliability of the PSI with extensive use with diverse samples of various ages and backgrounds. Reliability coefficients calculated for each subscale ranged from .70 to .84, and reliability coefficients for the Child and Parent Domains and Total Stress Scale were .90 or greater. Stability of the PSI is supported by test-retest coefficients ranging from .55 to .96 in studies using time intervals of 3 weeks to 1 year. Reliability estimates for the PSI/SF were comparable to those for the full-length version. Principal components analysis with varimax rotation produced three factors that comprise the PSI/SF subscales of parental distress, parent-child dysfunctional interaction, and difficult child. A total stress score also can be calculated (Abindin). The PSI/SF was used in this study because its short format reduces subject burden, and reliability and validity issues have been adequately addressed. Cronbach's alpha reliability estimate for the PSI/SF in this study was .925.

PROCEDURES

This study was a continuation of the larger "Baby Talk" project in which researchers examined the efficacy of an interactive coaching intervention to promote responsiveness between mothers with depressive symptoms and their infants (Horowitz et al., 2001). Prior to initiating the study, the researchers obtained Human Subject Committee approval from the university and clinical institutions.

Because the intervention had no effect on maternal depressive levels, combining treatment and control group participants was feasible for this follow-up study to examine long-term course of maternal depression symptoms. However, to insure that group assignment in the intervention study had no significant effect on depression symptom levels at 2 years postpartum, the investigators compared depression symptom means (EPDS and BDI-II scores) of women originally assigned to the treatment and control groups. No significant mean differences were found. Therefore, the groups were combined.

Mothers were recruited while they were patients on the postpartum units of a large teaching hospital in Boston and another hospital in southeastern Massachusetts. Postpartum nurses gave information about the study to English-speaking women who delivered healthy babies, defined as those infants discharged with a normal newborn exam. Women returned forms indicating permission to be contacted at 2 to 4 weeks to answer questions about how they were feeling emotionally. Research nurses contacted women who had given permission and administered the screening questionnaire by telephone, or they sent the questionnaire by mail after two failed attempts by phone. Women whose EPDS scores were 10 or higher were invited to participate in the study.

Research nurses visited participants in their homes when their babies were 4 to 8 weeks (Time 1), 10 to 14 weeks (Time 2), and 14 to 18 weeks old (Time 3). At each visit, research nurses evaluated mothers' depression scores and assisted mothers to contact their primary care providers for a clinical evaluation whenever their EPDS score was in the moderate to severe range. In this follow-up study, researchers contacted women approximately 2 years after delivery (Time 4) to examine the long-term course of depression symptoms.

PARTICIPANTS

Women who delivered at two hospitals in the northeastern United States, and who granted permission to be contacted after discharge for mental health screening, comprised the study population. Of the 1,215 women who completed the EPDS at

2 to 4 weeks postpartum, 123 women with elevated EPDS scores agreed to participate in the study. Of these, 117 completed the data collection phases through Time 3 (14-18 weeks postpartum). Sixty-two of these participants could be located and agreed to participate in the assessment at 2 years after delivery.

The mean age of women in the 2-year post-delivery sample was 33.6 years (range 21-43 years). Participants indicated their racial and ethnic designations as 74.2% European American/White, 3.2% Asian or Pacific Islander, 3.2% Hispanic, 1.6% Native American, 1.6% Middle Eastern, and 16.1% mixed or other. Eighty-seven percent of the women were married, and 93.5% were living with a partner. Fifty-six percent of the participants were primiparas. Yearly household income ranged from under $10,000 to over $90,000 with 31% of subjects having income less than $50,000 and 29% having income greater than $90,000. The sample was generally well educated. All participants had at least 2 years of college education, with an average of 16.7 years of education (*SD* = 2.8) and a range of 12 to 24 years. In comparison to the original sample, the 2-year postdelivery sample had a slightly higher percentage of Caucasian women, no African Americans, and a slightly lower percentage of Latinas; however, a higher percentage of women identified as having mixed race/ethnicity. The 2-year postdelivery sample also included a smaller percentage of first-time mothers than the original sample (i.e., 66% in the original sample vs. 56% in the follow-up sample). Otherwise, no appreciable differences between the two samples were noted.

ANALYSIS

Repeated measures analysis of variance (R-ANOVA) was used to answer Research Question 1. BDI-II scores were used for the depression symptom variable because these data were available at all time points from the original "Baby Talk" study (Horowitz et al., 2001) and, therefore, were obtained at 2-year follow-up. Before the R-ANOVA was performed, square root transformations of the BDI-II scores were performed to meet the assumption of normality of the distributions. The analysis included one within-subjects factor, depression symptoms, measured by the BDI-II, at four times: Times 1 through 4. Mauchley's test of sphericity was statistically significant, indicating that the assumption of compound symmetry was not met; therefore, the univariate results with the Greenhouse-Geisser epsilon correction are reported. Correlation analyses and hierarchical multiple regression were used to answer Research Question 2. The following factors were selected as potential predictors of depression scores at Time 4: maternal age, parity, income, depression history, Time 1 depression (i.e., baseline BDI-II score), overall support, and the following indicators of parenting stress: parental distress, parent-child dysfunctional interaction, and difficult child (i.e., PSI/SF subscales), and total parent stress (PSI/SF total score). These factors were selected for analysis because they were identified previously in the literature as important maternal descriptors and possible predictors of a more prolonged postpartum depression course.

RESULTS

Research Question 1 was answered as follows: At Time 4, 2 years after delivery, 30.6% of participants had BDI-II scores in the depressed range. The means, standard deviations, percentages of participants whose scores fell in the depressed range, and percentages for score categories across the four times are displayed in Table 3.1. There was a significant change in BDI-II scores over time (p = .001); however, pairwise comparisons indicated that the significant decrease in mean scores occurred from Time 1 to Time 2. BDI-II mean scores across Times 2, 3, and 4 did not differ significantly. Results are displayed in Table 3.2.

Research Question 2 was answered through the following analyses. Correlation analyses revealed that the following maternal factors were significantly related to depression scores at Time 4: parity, income, depression history, Time 1 BDI-II score (i.e., baseline depression), overall social support, and parental distress. Total parent stress (i.e., the combined scores from the PSI/SF subscales) also was positively correlated with Time 4 depression scores; however, among the subscales, only parental distress showed a positive relationship to depression. Correlations are displayed in Table 3.3. Factors with significant correlations to maternal depression at Time 4 were selected for inclusion in the subsequent analysis.

In the hierarchical multiple regression analysis, Set 1 of independent variables comprised parity, income, and depression history. These variables were entered first because they were preexisting factors from maternal history. Set 1 accounted for .291% of the variance (p = .001). Set 2 comprised baseline depression (Time 1 BDI-II scores) to evaluate the effect of early postpartum depression symptom severity. Set 2 added an additional 5.8% of variance (F change: p = .029). Set 3 comprised current (i.e., Time 4) situational variables of overall social support and parental distress. Set 3 added an additional 19.5% of variance (F change: p = .000). The three sets accounted for 54.4% of the variance in maternal depression scores at Time 4. In the final model, a positive depression history, lower overall support, and higher parental distress were significant predictors of maternal depression symptoms at Time 4. Results are displayed in Table 3.4.

TABLE 3.1. BDI-II Scores[a] at Times 1–4

Time	*M*	Standard Depressed	Total Depressed	Mildly Depressed (14-19)	Moderately Depressed (20-28)	Severely Depressed (29-63)
Time 1	14.12	7.34	41.9%	22.6%	14.5%	4.8%
Time 2	10.75	6.84	35.5%	24.2%	9.7%	1.6%
Time 3	10.65	6.87	27.4%	11.3%	16.1%	0.0%
Time 4	11.57	9.49	30.6%	16.1%	4.8%	9.7%

[a]Nontransformed scores are displayed.

TABLE 3.2. Repeated Measures Analysis of Variance for Maternal Depression Scores

Source of Variance	*SS*	*df*	*MS*	*F*	*p*
BDI-II scores over time[a]	9.27	1	9.27	13.67	.000*
Error	41.35	61	.68		

Note. SS = Type III Sum of Squares.
* = statistically significant result.
[a]Significant change from Time 1 to Time 2.

TABLE 3.3. Correlations Between Maternal Factors and Time 4 Maternal Depression Scores

	BDI-II Time 4	BDI-II Time 4 Transformed
Maternal age	.037 (p = .775)	.052 (p = .685)
Parity	.400 (p = .001)	.355 (p = .005)
Income	-.413 (p = .001)	-.402 (p = 001)
Depression history	.381 (p = .002)	.305 (p = .016)
Baseline depression	.608 (p = .000)	.584 (p = .000)
Overall support	-.401 (p = .001)	-.429 (p = .000)
Parental distress	.561 (p = .000)	.571 (p = .001)
Difficult child	.231 (p = .071)	.226 (p = .077)
Parent-child difficult interaction	.161 (p = .211)	.156 (p = .227)
Total parental stress	.425 (p = .001)	.430 (p = .001)

DISCUSSION

In this sample of at-risk women, as determined by elevated EPDS scores at 2 weeks postpartum, 30.6% were still experiencing depressive symptoms at approximately 2 years postpartum: 16.1% mild, 4.8% moderate, and 9.7% severe levels of symptoms. A significant decrease in depression scores during the postpartum period from 4 to 8 weeks to 10 to 14 weeks after delivery was detected. However, following this initial

TABLE 3.4. Hierarchical Regression Analysis for Variables Predicting Time 4 Maternal Depression Scores

Predictor Variables	*R*	R^2	R^2 Change	*F* of Equation	*B*	*SE*	β	Sig.
Step 1	.539	.291	.291	7.792				
Parity					.350	.194	.213	.077
Income					-.174	.059	-.341	.005
Depression history					.822	.396	.234	.043
Step 2	.591	.349	.058	7.51				
Parity					.280	.190	.170	.147
Income					-.140	.059	-.274	.021
Depression history					.548	.402	.158	.178
Baseline depression					.838	.374	.273	.029
Step 3	.738	.544	.195	10.747				
Parity					.161	.167	.098	.338
Income					-.084	.052	-.164	.113
Depression history					.749	.345	.216	.035
Baseline depression					.243	.345	.079	.484
Overall support					-.158	.074	-.221	.036
Parental distress					.074	.018	.423	.000

Note. Variables remaining in the final model: depression history, overall support, and parental distress.

decline in mean depression scores, no subsequent significant decrease over time was found. These findings confirm patterns detected by other investigators (Beeghly et al., 2002; Campbell & Cohn, 1997; Small et al., 1994) regarding timing of depression change and the tendency for depression to persist throughout and beyond the first postpartum year if a woman is depressed at 2 to 3 months postpartum.

The decrease in depression symptoms from Time 1 to Time 2 suggests that for many women, postpartum depression symptoms may be a time-limited problem with peak occurrence during early postpartum weeks. Yet the lack of significant decrease in depression scores on the BDI-II after Time 2 and the percentage of women who scored above the cutoff for depression scores on the BDI-II at Time 4 also indicated that symptoms persisted for many women. The longitudinal pattern of postpartum depression symptom scores demonstrated the usefulness of screening postpartum populations and tracking symptom levels over time to differentiate those women at risk for clinical depression who need psychotherapy and possibly psychopharmacologic treatment from those who would benefit from monitoring and less intensive supportive counseling interventions. The persistence of depressive symptoms for many women demonstrates the importance of continued evaluation of women whose depression symptoms remain elevated at 2 to 3 months postpartum. Thus, monitoring of postpartum depression severity and duration is needed in clinical practice and will be valuable in future research.

In this sample, women with a depression history, lower overall support, and higher parental stress were at increased risk for being depressed at 2 years after delivery compared with their counterparts. Findings confirm previous research outcomes that poor social support was associated with ongoing depression (Seguin et al., 1999), although lower income, another predictor identified in the literature (Hobfoll et al., 1995; Seguin et al.), dropped out as a predictor when overall support and parental distress were added to the model. In contrast to previously reported findings that prior history of depression was not associated with ongoing depression (Campbell & Cohn, 1997; Zelkowitz & Milet, 2001), depression history was a significant predictor. Furthermore, baseline depression also dropped out of the model as a predictor when overall support and parental distress were included in the model. This result fails to confirm outcomes reported by Beeghly and colleagues (2002) that mothers with higher depression scores at 2 months postpartum were at increased risk of continuing to experience high levels of symptoms throughout the first postpartum year. Perhaps the longer time frame in the current study accounts for this difference. Interestingly, neither child difficulty nor problematic mother-child relations predicted persistence of depressive symptoms, in contrast to previously reported research results (Campbell et al., 1995; Seguin et al.). Possibly many mothers in this study who experienced early postpartum depression symptoms were able to develop relatively positive outlooks on their mother-child interactions regardless of whether or not their depression symptoms persisted. On the other hand, observation of interactions might discern links between depression severity and impaired quality of the mother-child interaction that were not discerned by self-report measures. Nonetheless, parental distress did predict depression at 2 years postpartum, suggesting that current stress related to parenting is related to maternal depression symptoms.

Limitations of this study should be weighed when interpreting the results. The design excluded women who could not speak English, and sampling occurred only within southeastern New England. Conducting clinical interviews to determine diagnostic status and validation of depression scores was not feasible; thus, assessments of depressive symptoms were based only on self-report. The Time 4 sample size was just slightly more than half of the number from Times 1 through 3. Many participants from the original sample had changed addresses and were unable to be located for follow-up inclusion. The findings also were limited concerning subsequent pregnancies, childbirth, or other major life events among the women at Time 4 because these data were not collected. Such information may have provided possible explanations for the nonsignificant increase in depression scores from Time 3 to Time 4 in this sample, although the number of women who might have had another pregnancy or major life event within the time frame probably would have been too small to allow for such analysis.

Strengths of the study, however, enhance credibility of the results. Screening a large number of postpartum women produced a sample of participants with known postpartum depression symptoms (Horowitz et al., 2001). Follow-up assessments with a standardized depression measure enabled the researchers to track symptoms from postpartum to 2 years after delivery. To date, such longitudinal data are limited. Thus, these results contribute useful information about the long-term course of maternal depression symptoms and associated risk factors.

Clinical implications can be derived from the study's findings. The lack of significant changes in mean depression scores over time from 10 to 14 weeks and 14 to 18 weeks to 2 years after delivery indicates the need for long-term clinical follow-up of at-risk women. To prevent possible chronic depression and related negative effects on maternal and family health, ongoing clinical evaluation and treatment of postpartum women whose depression symptoms do not remit after the first few postpartum weeks are warranted. This study's results indicate the need to extend assessments beyond the first postpartum year at least through children's toddler period for women whose postpartum depression symptoms suggest vulnerability to ongoing depression.

Recommendations for routine screening of all postpartum women have been made previously (Georgiopoulos et al., 1999; Horowitz et al., 1996; Horowitz et al., 1995), although such recommendations are yet to be widely adopted. In the hospital settings involved in this study, postpartum depression screening occurred only if the obstetric providers incorporated mental health evaluation as part of routine postpartum follow-up care: such depression screening was not yet standard care.

Based on their assessments of postpartum depressive symptoms, Affonso and colleagues (2000) suggested that single-point assessments are inadequate and recommended assessment beyond the early postpartum weeks. Furthermore, this study's results support the need to extend evaluation of women who exhibit elevated depression symptoms at initial screening through the second postpartum year. Findings from this study also indicated that women who had experienced previous depression, who had limited social support, and who had experienced subjective parental distress were most in need of follow-up because they were at highest risk for chronic depression. Clinical evaluation of these factors is merited.

Research implications include the importance of conducting more investigations with longitudinal designs to discern depression patterns and risk factors for chronic depression. Investigations of parenting and protective factors among women with ongoing depression also are needed. Including non-English-speaking women and obtaining large representative samples are other laudable research goals to extend understanding of maternal depression associated with postpartum onset.

CONCLUSIONS

Symptom assessments over time demonstrated that approximately 30% of women identified as at-risk for depression through early screening exhibited ongoing elevated depression symptoms. These findings confirm the importance of identification and treatment of postpartum depression to prevent or mitigate potential instances of chronic depression among vulnerable women. A positive depression history, lower overall support, and higher parental stress were predictors of higher maternal depression scores at 2 years postpartum. Assessment of such maternal factors in practice at regularly scheduled health appointments could identify women who are at risk or who may be experiencing ongoing depression. Such regular evaluation also may offer avenues for intervention, including building in supportive peer experiences and parenting help. Thus, standardizing clinical appraisal of postpartum depression symptoms and implementing early intervention might reduce unremitting maternal depressions and possibly improve quality of life for mothers and their families. In addition, longitudinal research is needed to determine factors that increase or ameliorate risk for chronic maternal depression.

REFERENCES

Abindin, R. R. (1995). *Parenting stress index (3rd ed.): Professional manual.* Odessa, FL: Psychological Assessment Resources.

Affonso, D. D., De, A., Horowitz, J. A., & Mayberry, L. J. (2000). An international comparative study exploring postpartum depression symptoms. *Journal of Psychosomatic Research, 49*, 207-216.

Affonso, D. D., Lovett, S., Paul, S., Sheptak, S., Nussbaum, R., Newman, L., et al. (1992). Dysphoric distress in childbearing women. *Journal of Perinatology, 12*(4), 325-332.

Areias, M. E. G., Kumar, R., Barros, H., & Figueredo, E. (1996). Comparative incidence of depression in women and men during pregnancy and after childbirth. Validation of the Edinburgh Postnatal Depression Scale in Portuguese mothers. *British Journal of Psychiatry, 169*, 30-35.

Bagedahl-Strindlund, M., & Monsen Borjesson, K. (1998). Postnatal depression: A hidden illness. *Acta Psychiatrica Scandinavica, 98*, 272-275.

Ballard, C. G., Davis, R., Cullen, P. C., Mohan, R. N., & Dean, C. (1994). Prevalence of postnatal psychiatric morbidity in mothers and fathers. *British Journal of Psychiatry, 164*, 782-788.

Beck, A. T., Steer, R. A., & Brown, G. K. (1996). *BDI-II: 2nd Edition Manual.* San Antonio, TX: The Psychological Corporation.

Beck, A. T., Steer, R. A., & Garbin, M. G. (1988). Psychometric properties of the Beck Depression Inventory: Twenty-five years of evaluations. *Clinical Psychology Review, 8*, 77-100.

Beck, A. T., Ward, C. H., Mendelson, M., Mock, J., & Erbaugh, J. (1961). An inventory for measuring depression. *Archives of General Psychiatry, 4*, 561-569.

Beck, C. T. (1995). The effects of postpartum depression on maternal-infant interaction: A meta-analysis. *Nursing Research, 44*(5), 298-304.

Beck, C. T. (1996). A meta-analysis of predictors of postpartum depression. *Nursing Research, 45*, 297-303.

Beck, C. T. (1998). The effects of postpartum depression on child development: A meta analysis. *Archives of Psychiatric Nursing, 12*(1).

Beck, C. T. (2001). Predictors of postpartum depression. *Nursing Research, 50*, 275-285.

Beeghly, M., Weinberg, M. K., Olson, K. L., Kernan, H., Riley, J. M., & Tronick, E. Z. (2002). Stability and change in level of maternal depressive symptomatology during the first postpartum year. *Journal of Affective Disorders, 71*, 169-180.

Brennan, P. A., Hammen, C., Andersen, M. J., Bor, W., Najman, J. M., & Williams, G. M. (2000). Chronicity, severity, and timing of maternal depressive symptoms: Relationships with child outcomes at age 5. *Developmental Psychology, 36*(6), 759-766.

Brown, S., & Lumley, J. (2000). Physical health problems after childbirth and maternal depression at six to seven months postpartum. *BJOG: An International Journal of Obstetrics and Gynecology, 107*, 1194-1201.

Campbell, S. B., & Cohn, J. F. (1997). The timing and chronicity of postpartum depression: Implications for infant development. In L. Murray & P. J. Cooper (Eds.), *Postpartum depression and child development* (pp. 165-197). New York: The Guilford Press.

Campbell, S. B., Cohn, J. F., & Meyers, T. (1995). Depression in first-time mothers: Mother-infant interaction and depression chronicity. *Developmental Psychology, 31*(3), 349-357.

Cox, J. L., Holden, J. M., & Sagovsky, R. (1987). Detection of postnatal depression: Development of the 10-item Edinburgh Postnatal Depression Scale. *British Journal of Psychiatry, 150*, 782-786.

Deater-Deckard, K., Pickering, K., Dunn, J. F., & Golding, J. (1998). Family structure and depressive symptoms in men preceding and following the birth of a child: The Avon longitudinal study of pregnancy and childhood study team. *American Journal of Psychiatry, 155*(6), 818-823.

Evans, J., Heron, J., Francomb, H., Oke, S., & Golding, J. (2001). Cohort study of depressed mood during pregnancy and after childbirth. *British Medical Journal*, 323(7307), 257-260.

Field, T. (1995). Infants of depressed mothers. *Infant Behavior and Development, 18*, 1-13.

Georgiopoulos, A. M., Bryan, T. L., Yawn, B. P., Houston, M. S., Rummans, T. A., & Therneau, T. M. (1999). Population-based screening for postpartum depression. *Obstetrics and Gynecology, 93*, 653-657.

Hiscock, H., & Wake, M. (2001). Infant sleep problems and postnatal depression: A community-based study. *Pediatrics, 107*(6), 1317-1322.

Hobfoll, S. E., Ritter, C., Lavin, J., Hulsizer, M. R., & Cameron, R. P. (1995). Depression prevalence and incidence among inner-city pregnant and postpartum women. *Journal of Consulting and Clinical Psychology, 63*(3), 445-453.

Horowitz, J. A., Bell, M., Trybulski, J., Munro, B. H., Moser, D., Hartz, S., et al. (2001). Promoting responsiveness between mothers with depressive symptoms and their infants. *Journal of Nursing Scholarship, 33*(4), 323-329.

Horowitz, J. A., Damato, E., Solon, L., & von Metzsch, G. (1996). Identification of symptoms of postpartum depression: Linking research to practice. *Journal of Perinatology, 16*(5), 360-365.

Horowitz, J. A., Damato, E., Solon, L., Von Metzsch, G., & Gill, V. (1995). Postpartum depression: Issues in clinical assessment. *Journal of Perinatology, 15*(4), 268-278.

Josefsson, A., Berg, G., Nordin, C., & Sydsjo, G. (2001). Prevalence of depressive symptoms in late pregnancy and postpartum. *Acta Obstetricia Gynecologica Scandinavica, 80*, 251-255.

Lane, A., Keville, R., Morris, M., Kinsella, A., Turner, M., & Barry, S. (1997). Postnatal depression and elation among mothers and their partners: Prevalence and predictors. *British Journal of Psychiatry, 171*, 550-555.

Matthey, S., Barnett, B., Ungerer, J., & Waters, B. (2000). Paternal and maternal depressed mood during the transition to parenthood. *Journal of Affective Disorders, 60*(2), 75-85.

McIntosh, J. (1993). The experience of motherhood and the development of depression in the postnatal period. *Journal of Clinical Nursing, 2*, 243-249.

Miller, L. J. (2002). Postpartum depression. *Journal of the American Medical Association, 287*(6), 762-765.

Nielson, F. D., Videbech, P., Hedegaard, M., Dalby, S. J., & Secher, N. J. (2000). Postpartum depression: Identification of women at risk. *British Journal of Obstetrics and Gynecology, 107*, 1210-1217.

O'Hara, M. W., & Swain, A. M. (1996). Rates and risk of postpartum depression—A meta-analysis. *International Review of Psychiatry, 8*, 37-54.

Seguin, L., Potvin, L., St.-Denis, M., & Loiselle, J. (1999). Depressive symptoms in the late postpartum among low socioeconomic status women. *Birth, 26*(3), 157-163.

Sichel, D. (2000). Postpartum psychiatric disorders. In M. Steiner, K. Yonkers, & E. Eriksson (Eds.), *Mood disorders in women* (pp. 313-328). London: Martin Dunitz.

Small, R., Brown, S., Lumley, J., & Astbury, J. (1994). Missing voices: What women say and do about depression after childbirth. *Journal of Reproductive and Infant Psychology, 12*, 89-103.

Teti, D. M., Messinger, D. S., Gelfand, D. M., & Isabella, R. (1995). Maternal depression and the quality of early attachment: An examination of infants, preschoolers, and their mothers. *Developmental Psychology, 31*(3), 364-376.

Troutman, B., & Cutrona, C. (1990). Nonpsychotic postpartum depression among adolescent mothers. *Journal of Abnormal Psychology, 99*, 69-78.

Weinberg, M. K., Tronick, E. Z., Beeghly, M., Olson, K. L., Kernan, H., & Riley, J. M. (2001). Subsyndromal depressive symptoms and major depression in postpartum women. *American Journal of Orthopsychiatry, 71*(1), 87-97.

Whiffen, V. E., & Gotlib, I. H. (1993). Comparison of postpartum and nonpostpartum depression: Clinical presentation, psychiatric history, and psychosocial functioning. *Journal of Consulting and Clinical Psychology, 61*(3), 485-494.

Yonkers, K. A., Ramin, S. M., Rush, A. J., Navarrete, C. A., Carmody, T., March, D., et al. (2001). Onset and persistence of postpartum depression in an inner-city maternal health clinic system. *American Journal of Psychiatry, 158*(11), 1856-1863.

Zelkowitz, P., & Milet, T. H. (2001). The course of postpartum psychiatric disorders in women and their partners. *Journal of Nervous and Mental Disease, 189*(9), 575-582.

Acknowledgments. This research was supported in part by Research Grant 12-FY98-0014 from the March of Dimes Birth Defects Foundation, a Research Incentive Grant from Boston College, and a research grant from Alpha Chi Chapter, Sigma Theta Tau International. The authors acknowledge statistical consultation from Dr. Barbara Hazard Munro, PhD, FAAN, and Dr. Mary Duffy, PhD, FAAN; assistance of Bernadette Quigley-Lavoie, Nurse Manager Brigham and Women's Hospital (BWH), Boston, the nursing staffs and administrations of BWH and Brockton Hospital; and contributions of the "Baby Talk" study team and research assistants. We are indebted to all of the mothers who participated in the research project.

4

Prenatal Depression: A Randomized Controlled Trial in the Emotional Health of Primiparous Women

Barbara A. Hayes
Reinhold Muller

The incidence of postnatal depression is widely known in both popular and scientific literature, and the figures are relatively stable. From a synthesis of the prevalence of postnatal depression, Pope, Watts, Evans, McDonald, and Henderson state that "postnatal depression affects 12% to 15% of childbearing women, with prevalence varying from 3% to 30% depending on the method and time of assessment" (2000, p. 6). However, no such appreciation of the incidence of antenatal depression seems to be readily accessible.

As there have been fewer research studies on depression during pregnancy than postnatal depression, prevalence is more difficult to estimate accurately. This gap in the research literature attracted investigations into prenatal depression and its posited connection with postnatal depression since the early 1980s (Cox, Connor, & Kendell, 1982; Wolkind, Coleman, & Ghodisan, 1980). Although early research indicated that antenatal depression was less common or serious than postnatal depression (Cox et al., 1982), Pope and colleagues (2000) report that subsequent research suggests that the prevalence of unipolar depression during pregnancy ranges between 4% and 15% (Gotlib, Whiffen, Mount, & Cordy, 1989; Green & Murray, 1994; Kumar & Robson, 1984; O'Hara, Zekoski, & Philipps, 1990). Such prevalence rates indicate a significant problem for childbearing women, their families, and the clinicians who accompany them on the journey.

The same problems beset estimation of prevalence for prenatal depression as were experienced for postnatal depression—that is, prevalence for the same prenatal population can vary widely depending on the type of measurement employed for depressive symptoms, the most common being either self-report questionnaires (Condon & Corkindale, 1997) or confirmation of diagnosis of depression using standardized interview criteria (Cooper, Campbell, Day, Kennerley, & Bond, 1988; Gotlib et al., 1989; O'Hara, Stuart, Gorman, & Wenzel, 2000; O'Hara et al., 1990). Given these problems, then, researchers' interest in validation and confirmation of prevalence rates of prenatal depression can be appreciated.

During the hunt for predictors of postnatal depression, two meta-analyses identified a similar list of variables named as predictors of postnatal depression: O'Hara and Swain (1996) and Beck (1998). Beck reported on a previous meta-analysis of predictors of postpartum depression drawing on 84 studies conducted in the 1980s (Beck, 1995). Beck stated the following list to be postpartum depression predictors: social support, prenatal depression, life stress, marital relationship, depression history, infant temperament, socioeconomic status, childcare stress, self-esteem, unplanned/unwanted pregnancy, maternity blues, prenatal anxiety, and marital status. However, with a different perspective these 13 predictors of postnatal depression could be viewed as the profile of prenatal depression; some, of course, may be both. Take, for example, the following 4 "predictors": prenatal depression, prenatal anxiety, social support, and unplanned/unwanted pregnancy. These could well be the core profile of prenatal depression. Further, Lumley and Austin (2001) also report that postnatal psychological interventions, with very different theoretical bases, offered to women who had a depressive illness, were effective in only 50% of the cases. It may be possible that these women were still experiencing the effects of prenatal depression.

The history of rigorous measurement of depressive symptoms lies in the development of the Saint Louis Criteria (Feighner et al., 1972) and, also, in the Research Diagnostic Criteria (RDC; Spitzer, Endicott, & Robins, 1981), both of which provided the basis for the generation of the groundbreaking third edition of the *Diagnostic and Statistical Manual of Mental Disorders* (DSM-III; American Psychiatric Association, 1980). The Scale for Affective Disorders and Schizophrenia (SADS) was a direct outcome of the application of well-validated RDC criteria for a rigorous diagnostic interview in clinical practice. Affonso, Lovett, Paul, and Sheptak (1990) modified the SADS for use in the diagnosis of depression in perinatal women (SADS-M) by selecting only the 27 items that measured depression and ensured that physiological changes in pregnancy and symptoms of clinical depression are not confused. The items are all rated singly with no total, or overall, score. The strength of the SADS-M is that it provides the researcher and the clinician with a range of strongly validated items to indicate the severity of depressive symptoms. However, it has no subscales, so its 27 dimensional scales have each item standing alone.

A range of other instruments have also yielded useful measurements. Hayes, Muller, and Bradley (2001) reported the results of a prospective, randomized controlled trial of an education intervention for primiparous women ($N = 206$) using the Profile of Mood States (POMS) as an outcome measure of mood. The POMS is a well-validated, 65-item, 5-point adjective rating scale with the following six subscales of mood measurement; tension, depression, anxiety, fatigue, confusion, and vigor—which is negatively weighted (Condon & Corkindale, 1997; McNair, Lorr, & Droppleman, 1981). On the other hand, the Edinburgh Postnatal Depression Scale (EPDS), developed by Cox, Holden, and Sagovsky (1987) is one of the most widely used instruments to screen for postnatal depression as opposed to diagnosing for depression. The EPDS is a 10-item, women-friendly scale with scores from 0 to 30 but with the usual cutoff (or reportable) point being 13 or above and, now, has been validated for use prenatally as well as its original postnatal use (Cox, 1994). The EPDS has proved useful in large studies to detect both prenatal and postnatal depression but not to detect the severity of symptoms. For example, Evans, Heron, Francomb, Oke, and Golding (2001) reported from a large sample of women in the United Kingdom (N = 9028) that women scored higher on the EPDS at 32 weeks antenatally than 8 weeks postnatally.

Three further sources of evidence support the position that the connection between prenatal and postnatal depression may not be the most salient question to pose, but viewing them as separate entities may lead to better recognition and management of depression. The first is that risk factors for postnatal depression are usually already impacting on women during pregnancy (Buist & Barnett, 1995); thus, it is more logical, and more efficacious, to address both the factors and effects on women prenatally than simply seeing these factors as predictors of postnatal depression. The second is the complexity of classifying depression before and after giving birth. Brockington (2004), in a detailed review of publications in postnatal psychiatry over the previous 5 years, states that the current accepted nomenclature of having three postnatal psychiatric disorders (maternity blues, postnatal depression, and postnatal psychosis) is an oversimplification and that the range of disorders is much broader. The third is that Lumley and Austin (2001), in a comprehensive and useful review of 10 controlled trials of interventions for the reduction of postnatal depression published from July 2000 to June 2001, found that the interventions, despite the timing (in pregnancy, in labor, or some time after birth) were disappointing.

Lumley and Austin (2001) report on the following three major areas:

1. antenatal screening for postpartum depression,
2. primary prevention of postpartum depression, and
3. secondary prevention of postpartum depression.

Only primary prevention of postpartum depression will be reported here. Seven trials of antenatal interventions designed to reduce the prevalence of postnatal depression were published prior to 2000. The two earliest projects—one in the United States by Gordon, Kapostina, and Gordon (1985), and one in the United Kingdom by Elliott, Sanjack, and Leverton (1988)—were influential in shaping the interventions developed in subsequent studies, including the one being reported in this current article. Gordon and associates (1985) emphasized the importance of preparing for the life changes associated with pregnancy, birth, and becoming a mother, and implemented a group intervention with a strong anticipatory guidance component and a focus on practical support. It reported a marked difference in "emotional upsets" at 6 to 8 weeks postpartum and in parents "having problems at 6 months." Thus, despite the intervention, women were still emotionally troubled 6 months after birthing a baby.

On the other hand, Elliott and colleagues (1988) reported on women who were screened as "vulnerable." The women were allocated to group interventions including five prenatal and six postnatal sessions which ran from the fourth month of pregnancy to 6 months after the birth. No significant differences in depression or anxiety scores were found at 6 weeks or 6 months after birth between the randomized groups, and no participant met the criteria for probable depression after birth. This study was replicated in Australia in a well-designed randomized trial, but the Elliott and Leverton screening tool identified 58% of women as vulnerable and few parous women participated (Stamp, Williams, & Crowther, 1995). Again, the intervention appears to have made little difference in either study (Elliott et al., 1988; Stamp et al., 1995). However, if interventions have demonstrated little effect in reducing postnatal depression but postnatal depression is still lower than prenatal depression in those studies when women's mood states were measured both pre- and postnatally, other competing explanations need to be sought.

Thus the aims of this study were to

1. Test the core hypothesis that women who receive an educational intervention in the prepartum period will have a lower level (by at least 0.3 scores) of depressive symptoms in the 16- to 24-week postpartum period than those who do not receive an educational intervention;
2. Develop pre- and postnatal profiles of the severity of symptoms of depression using a rigorous instrument based on RDC; and
3. Compare the prenatal and postnatal profiles of severity of depressive symptoms.

METHODS

DESIGN

A prospective, randomized controlled trial of an education intervention to reduce postnatal depression was conducted at three sites in Australia enrolling a total of 184 primiparous women. The intervention consisted of an information booklet on postnatal depression and an audiotape of one woman's journey through postnatal clinical depression. Mood was assessed prenatally (12-28 weeks) and twice postnatally (8-12 weeks and 16-24 weeks) using the SADS-M. Demographic and social support data were also collected at enrollment.

SETTING AND PROCEDURE

The study was conducted at three sites from January 1994 to December 1996. All sites were publicly funded hospitals and provided geographical, socioeconomic, and follow-up care. One hospital (Site A) is situated in a provincial city in northeast tropical Australia; the other two hospitals (Sites B and C) are situated in the capital cities of two states in southern Australia; Site A was approximately 4,000 kilometres from the other sites, and Site B and C were 1,200 kilometers apart. Both Sites A and B served a broadly lower socioeconomic group of women than Site C. Australia has a semisocialized system of health care available to all Australians, but many women invest in private health insurance, just for the birthing event, so that they will have more choice about the birthing attendants and the context in which they birth. Thus, women who attend public hospitals in large urban or provincial areas are, often, from a lower socioeconomic background and are unable to afford private health insurance.

Approval from the Human Subjects Ethics Committees of each hospital was successfully obtained. The duty-of-care implicit in obtaining informed consent from the women participants was addressed through the implementation of protocols specific to each health care delivery service, which the women attended. In Site A, the women were referred back to the parent hospital through the social work department; in Site B, the women were referred to the psychiatric/medical registrar and then to the consultant psychiatrist; in Site C, the women were referred back to the parent hospital by means of consultation and assessment with the psychiatric liaison nurse. At all sites, once women were "discharged" from the parent hospital, they were referred to general medical practitioners as close to their place of residence as possible, if still requiring psychological care; these general medical practitioners can be accessed at no cost to the woman.

Experienced midwives, who were trained specifically as research assistants for this project, collected all the data at interview. The SADS data were obtained in a face-to-face interview between the research assistant and the study participant, which took from 45 to 90 minutes, both prenatally and postnatally.

Sampling

Inclusion and Exclusion Criteria. Only primiparous women were recruited to avoid any potential confounding effects from intrafamilial and interpersonal variables (e.g., presence of other children, learning bias, and the temperament of a previous child) that could be possible competing explanations for the presence of depressive symptomatology (Kumar & Robson, 1984). Only women with a high school level of literacy or higher were enrolled because the intervention included an information booklet. The following exclusion criteria were applied: First, the presence of any prior diagnosed depressive episode in the previous 12 months to ensure that women who already had the best predictor of postnatal depression, that is, a previous episode of clinical depression (Kumar & Robson, 1984), were excluded; second, non-English-speaking women were excluded, because only English language instruments were used; and third, Australian indigenous women were excluded, because the instruments had not been culturally adapted for this group. Women were recruited through specific participating clinics at each hospital by the midwives who conducted the subsequent interviews; each consecutive woman who met the inclusion criteria was approached. Refusal was less than 1% and, mainly, was based on the level of perceived inconvenience involved rather than on lack of interest in the study.

Size and Power Calculation. Initial SADS-M measurements from a pilot study on prepartum women resulted in expected mean estimates of between 0.8 and 1.2 for the single items with standard deviations ranging from 0.4 to 0.8. It was calculated that a sample size of 90 for each of the two groups would yield a power of 80% at a two-sided alpha level of 5% to find a difference of +/-0.3 between the intervention group and the control group as significant when a conservatively estimated common standard deviation of 0.7 was assumed. Allowing for a dropout of 10%, a sample size of 100 for each group was targeted.

Randomization. After informed consent was obtained, a total of 206 primiparous women were randomized and assigned to the intervention or the control group in a center-stratified and balanced way. The project manager (the only person responsible for the allocation to either group at the three sites and not involved in the data collection) sent each site a list of consecutive balanced allocations generated using the statistical package SPSS. The data collection kits, stamped with the series number, were then sent to the sites and the research assistants recruited women into each group without knowledge of the allocation until after the recruitment. Out of the 206 randomized women, 184 (94 in the control group and 90 in the intervention group) completed the study protocol, reflecting a participation percentage of 89.3%.

The sample in one site was drawn from a population where there is a cyclical turnover of residents due to transfers of families within the civil and military services. The 22 women who did not complete the study had moved from the area, with short notice, without leaving a forwarding contact. Therefore, it could be ascertained that all losses to follow-up occurred for reasons unrelated to their emotional health. Moreover, the 22 women who were not available for postpartum interviews did not differ from those who completed the questionnaires in respect to their initial mood profile, demographics, or social support variables. Consequently selection bias arising from the women lost to follow-up can be excluded.

INSTRUMENTS

In all recruited women, the descriptive profile of antenatal mood was generated from the SADS-M. The SADS-M is a 27-item questionnaire developed from RDC (Spitzer et al., 1981); each item is scored from 1 to 5 with a score of 3 and above considered to be significant. Affonso and associates (1990) modified this instrument with a sample of primiparas from the San Francisco Bay area (N = 200) in the US. The modification weighted those items, which are shared by both the physiological changes in pregnancy and clinical depression (e.g., Fatigue, Weight Gain, Weight Loss, Body Concern, and Indecisiveness—that is, difficulty in making a decision). The other items are as follow: dysphoric mood, quality of mood, mood association, worrying, guilt, negative evaluation of self, discouragement, suicidal tendencies, somatic anxiety, psychological anxiety, phobia, mental slow down, loss of interest, social withdrawal, anger, irritability, agitation, psychomotor retardation, and functioning impairment. The SADS is used extensively in depression research, interrater reliability for SADS depression symptoms has been 0.90 or above, and test-retest reliabilities have been reported to be approximately 0.78 (Affonso et al., 1990; Spitzer et al., 1981).

In addition, the Norbeck Social Support Questionnaire (NSSQ) was employed to measure social support (Norbeck, 1990). The NSSQ has been validated across several studies (Norbeck) and consists of two sections. Section one is a nine-part questionnaire that elicits information of the subject's personal network of friends and family. A method of scoring builds up the profile of the composition of that network, the degree of functional support given to the subject, the frequency of contact, and the categories of people that the research participant may have recently lost contact with, for example, siblings. Section 2 elicits the following demographics: age, educational level, religion, and ethnic identity. Norbeck, Lindsey, and Carrieri (1981) reported the reliability and validity parameters for the NSSQ. Reliabilities for each of the subscales were as follows: Affect = 0.97; Affirmation = 0.96; Aid =

0.89. Rest-retest reliability correlations were as follows: Affect = 0.89; Affirmation = 0.88; Aid = 0.86. Similar high correlations were found for the three network properties, which were each 0.92. However, the authors reported only moderate concurrent validity and weak construct validity.

Further demographic data were obtained by means of another standardized questionnaire (Hayes, Oriti, & Hingst, 1994); the questions were developed from standard demographic tools and tested with experienced midwives. These data were collected once only.

Education Intervention

The education package was based on the work of Hillier and Slade (1989), who reported the beneficial effects of antenatal education in knowledge, anxiety, and confidence in primiparous women in the United Kingdom, and also on the established efficacy of education interventions in family interactions research in major mental disorders (Falloon, Boyd, & McGill, 1984). The package consisted of an information booklet designed and piloted for pregnant women, their partners, and extended family; a studio-quality audiotape of one woman's journey through postnatal clinical depression and back again; and an experienced midwife to guide the women through the package. The booklet contained six categories of information. First was the history of mood changes in childbearing women and an exploration of the range of names for the mood changes in plain English. The second category included information about some of the existing theories of the cause of mood change and the prevalence rates of mood changes in childbearing women among different cultures. The third category was information about the range of symptoms reported by women and, also, the intensity and frequency of those symptoms. The fourth offered guidelines about when, how, and where to seek assistance (tailored specifically to each site). The fifth outlined how each woman could develop a practical personal plan to seek and gain assistance if required. The sixth category offered information targeted specifically towards partners, extended family members, and friends. The women were interviewed by the same midwife research-assistant at all data collection points.

Statistical Analysis

Data were entered into a spreadsheet and submitted to thorough data cleaning processes. The numerical items of the Norbeck questionnaire proved to have a skewed distribution and, therefore, medians were used as measures of central tendency and quartiles as estimates of dispersion. Tests of these items between the two groups were conducted using exact versions of the unpaired nonparametric Wilcoxon tests. Categorical items of the Norbeck questionnaire between the groups were analyzed by exact versions of chi-square tests for nominal variables or chi-square tests for trend if the underlying item was of an ordinal structure.

Univariate analyses of the SADS-M variables revealed no evidence that the distributions of these numerical variables could not be assumed to follow a normal distribution. Consequently, univariate statistics are displayed as means (+/- standard deviations), and bivariate tests were performed using unpaired (control/intervention comparisons) and paired (pre/post comparisons) versions of the *t* tests. Multivariate regression analyses, using transformations of nonnormally distributed variables, were applied to check for potential confounding effects of demographics or social support variables. The adjusted multivariate findings were identical to the bivariate results disproving the presence of any confounding from the analyzed variables. Consequently, only bivariate results are displayed. For all tests, a *p*-value below 0.05 was regarded as significant, but this level of significance has to be interpreted cautiously since many tests were performed that could result in an inflation of Type I error.

RESULTS

Check of Randomization

Table 4.1 compares the demographic and the social support variables as measured by the Norbeck questionnaire between the two randomized groups. The first three data columns of Table 4.2 compare the prebirth measurements for the single SADS-M variable in both groups. It can be gathered from these tables that the randomization process was successful in that the two groups at baseline (prebirth) did not differ significantly in any of the social support variables and in only one item of the SADS-M variables: A difference in "guilt" was observed. This does not seem to have any potential to distort the reported findings since, taking the alpha level of 5% into account, even two "false-positive" test results (1 out of 20) would have been expected by chance alone. The randomization therefore proved successful.

Intervention

The second part of Table 4.2 lists the data relevant for assessing the intervention: The changes in mood (postnatal measurements at weeks 16-24 minus prenatal data at weeks 12-28) between the control and the intervention group are detailed. Not a single item on the SADS-M questionnaire showed a significant difference between the groups. That is, the educational intervention did not show any effect at all when the women's mood was measured by the SADS-M. Therefore, the core hypothesis, that women who receive an educational intervention in the prepartum period have a significantly lower level (by at least 0.3 scores) of depressive symptoms in the 16- to 24-week postpartum period than women without this intervention, has to be rejected. The identical results hold if the mood profile at postnatal weeks 8 to 12 is used as the outcome (data not displayed). Additional multivariate regression analyses revealed no relevant influence of social support or demographic variables in either group on the changes in mood.

Pre- and Postnatal Profiles of Mood

Table 4.3 specifies the prepartum and postpartum emotional health profiles of primiparous women. Since the intervention did not show any effect, data are presented for the entire sample (i.e., intervention and control group together). The general, substantial trend is that women are less depressed at weeks 8 to 12 postnatally than prenatally and that their profile of mood improves even further when measured at weeks 16 to 24 postnatally.

TABLE 4.1. Control of Randomization: Comparisons of Demographics and Norbeck Social Support Scales

	Control Group (n = 94)		Interv. Group (n = 90)		p-Value
Age	26	(23-30)	25	(23-29)	0.39
Norbeck (Affection 1)	28	(22-37)	31	(22-37)	0.77
Norbeck (Affection 2)	26	(20-39)	31	(20-38)	0.32
Norbeck (Affirmation 1)	26	(21-34)	27	(20-35)	0.60
Norbeck (Affirmation 2)	25	(19-32)	28	(20-36)	0.25
Norbeck (Aid 1)	25	(20-36)	28	(20-39)	0.46
Norbeck (Aid 2)	21	(17-29)	23	(19-33)	0.13
Norbeck (Duration)	28	(22-38)	31	(23-40)	0.49
Norbeck (Frequency)	27	(21-34)	27	(20-36)	0.57
Site					0.68
Townsville	27.4%		22.2%		
Melbourne	28.7%		32.2%		
Adelaide	43.6%		45.6%		
Religion					0.27
Religious	63.8%		72.2%		
Non-religious	36.2%		27.8%		
Religious Participation					0.58
Inactive/non-relig.	68.1%		57.8%		(trend test)
Irregular	20.3%		34.4%		
Regular	11.7%		7.8%		
Marital Status					0.57
Couple	79.8%		83.8%		
Single	20.2%		16.7%		
Ethnicity					0.77
Caucasian	92.6%		94.4%		
Other	7.4%		5.6%		
Education Level					0.23
Up to Grade 12	59.6%		49.4%		(trend test)
TAFE attempt/compl.	19.1%		24.1%		
Uni attempt/compl.	21.3%		26.4%		

Note. Displayed are medians and 25%-75% percentiles for numerical variables and percentages for categorical variables. p-values refer to comparisons between the groups (unpaired nonparametric Wilcoxon test for numerical and exact versions of unpaired chi-square tests or chi-square tests for trend for categorical variables). TAFE = Technical and Further Education College.

Women's improvement of mood is evidenced by a significant reduction in the vast majority of the items. Discouragement, anxiety, anger, irritability, and psychomotor retardation also all show a trend for improvement, though not reaching significance. The "positive" sign of weight loss is self-explanatory. Only with respect to the subscales of appetite loss and body concern, no clear trend was observable.

TABLE 4.2. Control of Randomization and Test of Intervention

	Control of Randomization					Test of Intervention Δ = (wks 12-28 pre)-(wks 16-24 post)				
SASD-M Variable	Control Group Prenatal n = 94		Interv. Group Prenatal n = 90		p-Value	Change in Control Group n = 94		Change in Interv. Group n = 90		p-Value
234 Dysphoric Mood	1.91 (0.87)	8	1.76 (0.77)	1	0.22	-0.33 (1.20)	8	-0.21 (0.87)	2	0.45
236 Qual. Of Mood	1.84 (1.08)	14	1.82 (0.94)	18	0.91	-0.13 (1.33)	34	-0.48 (1.06)	29	0.12
237 Mood Assoc.	1.57 (0.89)	32	1.65 (0.82)	30	0.58	-0.15 (0.99)	53	-0.37 (0.99)	44	0.30
238 Worrying	2.12 (1.00)	4	1.91 (0.79)	1	0.12	-0.34 (1.19)	5	-0.11 (0.93)	2	0.16
240 Guilt	1.47 (0.64)	2	1.28 (0.50)	0	0.026	-0.27 (0.79)	2	-0.11 (0.68)	1	0.15
242 Neg. Evaluation	1.57 (0.75)	4	1.57 (0.69)	0	1.00	-0.11 (1.02)	12	-0.21 (0.73)	3	0.48
244 Discouragement	1.30 (0.51)	5	1.34 (0.57)	2	0.64	+0.05 (0.63)	7	-0.06 (0.78)	2	0.34
246 Suic. Tendencies	1.11 (0.38)	2	1.11 (0.31)	11	0.98	-0.07 (0.44)	2	-0.10 (0.34)	9	0.58
263 Somatic Anxiety	1.46 (0.70)	2	1.38 (0.67)	1	0.25	-0.21 (0.78)	3	-0.12 (0.96)	3	0.47
265 Psych. Anxiety	1.46 (0.70)	2	1.38 (0.57)	1	0.44	-0.08 (0.96)	2	-0.07 (0.82)	1	0.95
269 Phobia	1.95 (0.94)	1	1.81 (0.91)	0	0.32	-0.23 (0.93)	4	-0.28 (0.97)	0	0.75
275 Insomnia	1.82 (0.85)	2	1.80 (0.90)	2	0.88	-0.43 (0.94)	4	-0.40 (1.10)	2	0.82
314 Sleeping more	2.04 (1.23)	2	2.03 (1.25)	2	0.96	-0.76 (1.34)	4	-0.65 (1.55)	2	0.62
315 Fatigue	1.97 (0.95)	2	2.01 (0.89)	0	0.75	-0.33 (1.12)	3	-0.42 (1.02)	1	0.59
317 Appetite Loss	1.29 (0.64)	3	1.23 (0.58)	1	0.50	+0.02 (0.93)	4	+0.06 (0.94)	4	0.80
319 Weight Loss	1.14 (0.41)	13	1.14 (0.67)	10	0.99	+0.55 (1.22)	36	+0.63 (1.40)	25	0.74
320 Appetite Increase	1.69 (0.80)	2	1.84 (1.09)	2	0.27	-0.23 (1.17)	2	-0.33 (1.31)	3	0.57
322 Body Concern	1.28 (0.52)	2	1.35 (0.52)	1	0.40	+0.07 (0.80)	2	+0.01 (0.79)	1	0.65
324 Indecisiveness	1.48 (0.76)	1	1.39 (0.65)	0	0.36	-0.23 (0.86)	1	-0.19 (0.69)	0	0.75
325 Mental Slow Down	1.49 (0.67)	2	1.52 (0.72)	0	0.75	-0.11 (0.86)	3	-0.23 (0.81)	0	0.32
326 Loss of Interest	1.40 (0.58)	5	1.34 (0.50)	4	0.41	-0.18 (0.68)	9	-0.09 (0.63)	5	0.41
328 Social Withdrawal	1.34 (0.62)	1	1.32 (0.62)	0	0.81	-0.17 (0.72)	1	-0.11 (0.74)	0	0.57
330 Anger	1.80 (1.01)	3	1.67 (0.77)	1	0.34	-0.09 (1.13)	3	-0.09 (0.97)	1	0.99

332 Irritability	1.77	(0.81)	4	1.82	(0.71)	0	0.63	-0.07	(1.09)	5	-0.20	(0.93)	0	0.38
334 Agitation	1.39	(0.76)	4	1.29	(0.59)	1	0.34	-0.17	(0.74)	4	-0.10	(0.71)	2	0.55
342 Psychomot. Retard.	1.19	(0.39)	2	1.14	(0.34)	1	0.36	-0.08	(0.54)	2	-0.05	(0.50)	1	0.69
465 Funct. Impairment	1.22	(0.44)	11	1.16	(0.37)	4	0.39	-0.12	(0.58)	12	-0.12	(0.45)	6	0.97

Note. Displayed are means and (standard deviations) followed by the number of missing observations. Data column 3 lists p-values of comparisons of the prepartum baseline measurements between control and intervention group using unpaired t tests (Control of Randomization). Data column 6 lists p-values of unpaired t tests comparing the changes of mood (first vs. third measurement) of the SADS-M variables between the control and the intervention group (Test of Intervention).

TABLE 4.3. Emotional Health Profile of Primiparous Women at 12-28 Weeks Prepartum, at 8-12 Weeks Postpartum, at 16-24 Weeks Postpartum and Changes Between the First and Last Measurements

SADS-M Variable Total Sample n = 184	Prenatal Mood wks 12-28 pre			Postnatal Mood wks 8-12 post			Postnatal Mood wks 16-24 post			Change in Mood wks 12-28 pre vs. wks 16-24 post			Change p-Values
234 Dysphoric Mood	1.84	(0.82)	9	1.69	(0.82)	6	1.57	(0.72)	1	-0.26	(1.04)	10	0.001
236 Qual. Of Mood	1.83	(1.0)	32	1.74	(0.97)	50	1.41	(0.81)	44	-0.31	(1.21)	63	0.006
237 Mood Assoc.	1.61	(0.86)	62	1.29	(0.66)	75	1.23	(0.55)	73	-0.26	(0.99)	97	0.015
238 Worrying	2.02	(0.91)	5	1.82	(0.81)	3	1.77	(0.86)	2	-0.23	(1.07)	7	0.005
240 Guilt	1.37	(0.58)	2	1.30	(0.68)	2	1.18	(0.48)	1	-0.19	(0.74)	3	0.001
242 Neg. Evaluation	1.57	(0.72)	4	1.43	(0.76)	7	1.41	(0.70)	11	-0.16	(0.88)	15	0.020
244 Discouragement	1.32	(0.54)	7	1.23	(0.50)	6	1.31	(0.58)	4	-0.01	(0.71)	9	0.92
246 Suic. Tendencies	1.11	(0.35)	8	1.09	(0.37)	7	1.03	(0.20)	3	-0.08	(0.40)	11	0.008
263 Somatic Anxiety	1.44	(0.69)	3	1.31	(0.64)	2	1.28	(0.66)	3	-0.16	(0.87)	6	0.013
265 Psych. Anxiety	1.42	(0.64)	3	1.36	(0.69)	1	1.34	(0.66)	0	-0.07	(0.90)	3	0.282
269 Phobia	1.88	(0.93)	1	1.62	(0.80)	3	1.63	(0.78)	3	-0.26	(0.95)	4	0.001
275 Insomnia	1.81	(0.87)	4	1.44	(0.77)	4	1.41	(0.65)	2	-0.42	(1.02)	6	0.001
314 Sleeping more	2.04	(1.24)	4	1.18	(0.57)	6	1.35	(0.76)	2	-0.70	(1.44)	6	0.001
315 Fatigue	1.99	(0.92)	2	1.52	(0.79)	2	1.62	(0.78)	2	-0.37	(1.07)	4	0.001
317 Appetite Loss	1.26	(0.61)	4	1.51	(0.99)	6	1.29	(0.73)	4	+0.04	(0.93)	8	0.570
319 Weight Loss	1.14	(0.55)	23	2.12	(1.59)	6	1.74	(1.26)	51	+0.59	(1.31)	61	0.001
320 Appetite Increase	1.76	(0.95)	4	1.58	(1.01)	5	1.48	(0.87)	1	-0.28	(1.24)	5	0.003
322 Body Concern	1.32	(0.52)	3	1.32	(0.54)	4	1.35	(0.61)	0	+0.04	(0.79)	3	0.512
324 Indecisiveness	1.44	(0.71)	1	1.32	(0.60)	2	1.23	(0.53)	0	-0.21	(0.78)	1	0.001
325 Mental Slow Down	1.51	(0.70)	2	1.33	(0.60)	3	1.33	(0.64)	1	-0.17	(0.84)	3	0.006
326 Loss of Interest	1.37	(0.54)	9	1.34	(0.64)	6	1.24	(0.47)	5	-0.14	(0.65)	14	0.008
328 Social Withdrawal	1.33	(0.61)	1	1.24	(0.58)	2	1.20	(0.43)	0	-0.14	(0.73)	1	0.009
330 Anger	1.74	(0.90)	4	1.71	(0.93)	3	1.65	(0.91)	0	-0.09	(1.05)	4	0.259
332 Irritability	1.79	(0.76)	4	1.73	(0.78)	3	1.65	(0.78)	1	-0.13	(1.01)	5	0.077

334 Agitation	1.34	(0.68)	5	1.29	(0.68)	3	1.23	(0.56)	1	-0.14	(0.73)	6	0.014
342 Psychomot. Retard.	1.16	(0.37)	3	1.07	(0.28)	4	1.10	(0.36)	0	-0.06	(0.52)	3	0.116
465 Funct. Impairment	1.19	(0.41)	15	1.13	(0.44)	10	1.07	(0.27)	5	-0.12	(0.51)	18	0.003

Note. "Changes" were calculated as postnatal minus prenatal measurements, that is, a negative sign implies improvement except for items 317 and 319. Displayed are means and (standard deviations) followed by the number of missing observations; data column 5 lists p-values of paired t tests comparing profiles of mood at weeks 12-28 prenatal and at weeks 16-24 postnatal.

Multivariate regression analyses revealed no relevant influence of social support or demographic variables on the changes in mood.

Table 4.4 states the percentages (and actual numbers) of women who were "clinically significant," that is, scored 3 or above in the respective SADS-M items (a) prepartum (weeks 12-28) (b) postpartum (weeks 16-24), and (c) those who were clinically significant at both measurements. For example, 19.7% (*n* = 35) of women were suffering from clinically significant insomnia before giving birth, which compares to 5.1% (*n* = 9) having this problem after birth, and 1.7% (*n* = 3) were clinically significant both pre- and postpartum. That is, out of 35 women who suffered clinically significant insomnia before birth, 32 did not experience this problem after birth, but another 6 women experienced insomnia after birth and 3 women suffered from it before and after birth. As can be gathered from the last column of Table 4.4, this reduction in insomnia was statistically significant. The main trend of clinically significant distress is towards improvement when postpartum data are compared to prepartum measurements. All significant findings, again, reveal less distress postpartum. The increase of those suffering from "weight loss" is again quite self-explanatory. When compared to the results of Table 4.3, fewer items were found to improve statistically significantly, which is a reflection of the fact that this analysis used only dichotomized, that is, "reduced" information (clinically significant yes/no) as opposed to the analysis of Table 4.3, which was based on the full numerical measurement information.

DISCUSSION

The randomization process proved successful as the women in both groups reflected no relevant differences with respect to their demographics and their social support variables as measured by the Norbeck questionnaire, and only minimal differences in their reported mood profile on the 27 items when their mood was assessed during pregnancy. Both groups were similar in level of education in that approximately half of each group completed high school and half possessed post-high school qualifications; this demographic reflects balanced randomization of the groups and also demonstrates that socioeconomic status could not have any confounding potential. Other potential confounders also proved to be of no relevance in multivariate analyses. While women in the study attended maternal child heath nurses and general medical practitioners for baby-related problems, check-ups, and immunization postnatally, few women reported any alternate therapies for mood during the study. Reasons for loss to follow-up could be ascertained as moving out of the area and, thus, independent of the outcome, that is, the profile of mood. Therefore, the potential for selection bias arising from the women lost to follow-up is extremely small. As a consequence, the results as presented can be regarded as unbiased—that is, valid.

These results demonstrate three major findings. The first finding relates to the core hypothesis that the education intervention apparently had no effect—thus it was rejected. This finding is corroborated by reports by Lumley and Austin (2001), who

TABLE 4.4. Clinically Significant Women at 12-28 Weeks Prenatally, at 16-24 Weeks Postnatally, and at Both Points in Time

SASD-M Variable	*N*	Prenatally	Postnatally	Both Times	*p*-Value
234 Dysphoric Mood	174	15.5% (27)	9.8% (17)	3.4% (6)	0.11
236 Qual. Of Mood	121	18.2% (22)	10.7% (13)	2.5% (3)	0.13
237 Mood Assoc.	87	12.6% (11)	4.6% (4)	0.0% (0)	0.12
238 Worrying	177	23.7% (42)	18.1% (32)	8.5% (15)	0.17
240 Guilt	181	3.9% (7)	2.8% (5)	0.0% (0)	0.77
242 Neg. Evaluation	169	7.1% (12)	7.1% (12)	3.6% (6)	1.00
244 Discouragement	175	3.4% (6)	5.1% (9)	0.6% (1)	0.58
246 Suic. Tendencies	173	1.2% (2)	0.6% (1)	0.0% (0)	0.98
263 Somatic Anxiety	178	11.2% (20	5.6% (10)	1.1% (2)	0.08
265 Psych. Anxiety	181	7.2% (13)	8.3% (15)	1.1% (2)	0.84
269 Phobia	180	20.0% (36)	12.8% (23)	5.6% (10)	0.055
275 Insomnia	178	19.7% (35)	5.1% (9)	1.7% (3)	< 0.001
314 Sleeping more	178	30.3% (54)	8.4% (15)	2.2% (4)	< 0.001
315 Fatigue	180	23.9% (43)	11.7% (21)	5.0% (9)	0.002
317 Appetite Loss	176	5.1% (9)	7.4% (13)	0.6% (1)	0.50
319 Weight Loss	123	2.4% (3)	21.1% (26)	1.6% (2)	< 0.001
320 Appetite Increase	179	16.8% (30)	12.8% (23)	3.9% (7)	0.34
322 Body Concern	181	2.8% (5)	7.2% (13)	0.0% (0)	0.09
324 Indecisiveness	183	11.5% (21)	3.8% (7)	1.1% (2)	0.007
325 Mental Slow Down	181	10.5% (19)	7.2% (13)	2.2% (4)	0.31
326 Loss of Interest	170	1.8% (3)	1.8% (3)	0.6% (1)	1.00
328 Social Withdrawal	183	5.5% (10)	1.1% (2)	0.0% (0)	0.04
330 Anger	180	17.8% (32)	17.8% (32)	7.2% (13)	1.00
332 Irritability	179	14.5% (26)	14.0% (25)	3.4% (6)	0.98
334 Agitation	178	6.7% (12)	3.9% (7)	0.6% (1)	0.33
342 Psychomot. Retard.	181	0.0% (0)	1.1% (2)	0.0% (0)	0.50
465 Funct. Impairment	166	0.6% (1)	0.6% (1)	0.0% (0)	1.00

Note. Displayed are the number of paired observations (*N*) and the percentages (and number) of clinically significant women (i.e., with a score of 3 or above). *P*-values refer to exact versions of the paired McNemar test.

reviewed 10 published controlled trials of interventions, including 2 with substantial updates of earlier studies, but none of these studies has used the SADS-M. The SADS-M, based on RDC, is a robust instrument; admittedly, it is probably too long to use as a screening tool but, clinically, it has a long history of reliability and validity for the detection and diagnosis of depression. That the education intervention was not significant with such a robust measure of mood is open to several explanations. The most obvious one is that the education intervention was simply not of sufficient duration or substance to reduce postnatal levels of depression. A second possible explanation is that the education intervention may have been effective, in measurable terms, for a different dependent variable such as "Women Seeking Professional Help for Depressive Symptoms." A third explanation, and one favored by the authors, is the fact that the ineffective education intervention, when using a robust measure of mood such as the SADS-M, can be considered as contributing further evidence to the prenatal period being a separate entity to the postnatal period, with distinctive psycho-neuro-endocrine pathways. This last explanation challenges the previous perspective in the following ways; (a) that education in the prenatal period will endure into the postnatal period, and (b) that the prenatal period requires predominantly physiological monitoring rather than an equal emphasis on monitoring of psychological, emotional, and mental states.

The second finding is that the profile of symptoms experienced by pregnant women, when measured with a rigorous instrument based on RDC, displayed a level of severity not usually reported. The profile of mood reported by 184 primiparas during pregnancy is one of concern including, as it does, not only anxiety and dysphoric mood but also suicidal tendencies. Beck and Gable (2000, 2001) reported prenatal depression and anxiety as predictors of postnatal depression, but this study brings attention to prenatal anxiety and depression as being salient aspects of the profile of the mood of pregnant women which ought, in their own right, to attract the attention of clinicians and researchers. Importantly, the results also provide evidence that some women experience symptoms of anxiety and depression both pre- and postnatally.

However, if the second finding reflected the severity of symptoms for primiparous women, the third finding showed a continued trend towards reduction of severity when measured twice postnatally. As this result was common to both groups, attention is drawn towards what the groups shared rather than what was different: the experience of pregnancy and birth and, also, three interviews with the same midwife. Two possible explanations are that perinatal depression may have a natural trajectory of gradual reduction of symptom severity or that the three interviews, when women's mood was measured by SADS-M, were, in themselves, a positive intervention resulting in a reduction in negative mood.

Whatever the explanations, the implications for nurses and midwives caring for childbearing women are clear. First, the transfer of this knowledge provides evidence for a refocusing of practice in caring for pregnant women. All pregnant women need to be screened, by measurement, for prenatal anxiety and depression as well as for postnatal anxiety and depression much as nurses and midwives already screen these same women with measurements of the vital signs as an essential part of the physiological assessment of women pre- and postnatally. Second, reliance on prenatal education classes to ensure women's preparation for the immediate and midterm postnatal period needs to be reviewed. Not only has the major transition of birthing a child taken place between the pre- and postnatal periods, but the knowledge needed for prepartum emotional and mental health is probably not the same as the knowledge needed for postpartum mental health.

In conclusion, screening women prepartum will not predict postnatal depression but will detect prepartum depression and opens the opportunity for effective treatment and management. While much contemporary research (Beck, 1998; Buist, Westley & Hill, 2001; Meager & Milgrom, 1996; Milgrom, Martin & Negri, 1999) presents evidence for the deleterious effects on the child of a depressed mother, little is known of the deleterious effects of a depressed mother on the embryo and fetus. Further, any intervention needs to be tailored to the individual to be effective (Lumley & Austin, 2001), rather than having a standard intervention. In the light of this knowledge, and given the contemporary reality that nurses and midwives are often the primary health carers for pregnant and postnatal women, there is also an ethical imperative to transfer and apply this knowledge to current nursing and midwifery care of childbearing women.

REFERENCES

Affonso, D., Lovett, S., Paul, S., & Sheptak, S. (1990). A standardized interview that differentiates pregnancy and postpartum symptoms from perinatal clinical depression. *Birth, 17,* 121-130.

American Psychiatric Association. (1980). *Diagnostic and statistical manual of mental disorders* (3rd ed.). Washington, DC: Author.

Beck, C. T. (1995). The effects of postpartum depression on maternal-infant interaction: A meta-analysis. *Nursing Research, 44,* 298-304.

Beck, C. T. (1998). The effects of postpartum depression on child development: A meta-analysis. *Archives of Psychiatric Nursing, 12,* 12-20.

Beck, C. T., & Gable, R. K. (2000). Postpartum depression screening scale: Development and psychometric testing. *Nursing Research, 49,* 272-282.

Beck, C. T., & Gable, R. K. (2001). Further validation of the Postpartum Depression screening scale. *Nursing Research, 50,* 155-164.

Brockington, I. (2004). Postpartum psychiatric disorders. *Lancet, 363,* 303-310.

Buist, A., & Barnett, B. (1995). Childhood sexual abuse: A risk factor for postpartum depression? *Australian and New Zealand Journal of Psychiatry, 32,* 479-487.

Buist, A., Westley, D., & Hill, C. (1998). Antenatal prevention of postpartum depression. *Archives of Women's Health, 1,* 167-173.

Condon, J. T., & Corkindale, C. J. (1997). The assessment of depression in the postnatal period: A comparison of four self-report questionnaires. *Australian and New Zealand Journal of Psychiatry, 31,* 353-359.

Cooper, P. J., Campbell, E. A., Day, A., Kennerley, H., & Bond, A. (1988). Non-psychotic psychiatric disorder after childbirth: A prospective study of prevalence, incidence, course and nature. *British Journal of Psychiatry, 152,* 799-806.

Cox, J. L., Holden, J. M., & Sagovsky, R. (1987). Detection of postnatal depression. Development of the 10-item Edinburgh Postnatal Depression scale. *British Journal of Psychiatry, 150,* 782-786.

Cox, J. L., Connor, Y., & Kendell, R. E. (1982). Prospective study of the psychiatric disorders of childbirth. *British Journal of Psychiatry, 140,* 111-117.

Cox, J. (1994). *Perinatal psychiatry: Use and misuse of the Edinburgh Postnatal Depression Scale.* London: Gaskell.

Elliott, S. A., Sanjack, M., & Leverton, T. J. (1988). Parents' groups in pregnancy: A preventive intervention for postnatal depression? In B. Gottlieb (Ed.), *Marshalling social support: Formats, processes and effects* (pp. 87-110). London: Sage.

Evans, J., Heron, J., Francomb, H., Oke, S., & Golding, J. (2001). Cohort study of depressed mood during pregnancy and after childbirth. *British Medical Journal, 323,* 256-260.

Feighner, J. P., Robins, E., Guze, S. B., Woodruff, B. A., Winokur, G., & Munoz, R. (1972). Diagnostic criteria for use in psychiatric research. *Archives of General Psychiatry, 26,* 57-63.

Falloon, I. R. H., Boyd, J. L., & McGill, C. W. (1984). *Family care of schizophrenia: A problem-solving approach to the treatment of mental illness.* New York: Guilford.

Gordon, R. E., Kapostina, E. E., & Gordon, K. K. (1985). Factors in postpartum emotional adjustments. *Obstetrics and Gynaecology, 25,* 158-166.

Gotlib, I. H., Whiffen, V. E., Mount, J. H., & Cordy, N. I. (1989). Prevalence rates and demographic characteristics associated with depression in pregnancy and the postpartum. *Journal of Consulting and Clinical Psychology, 57,* 269-274.

Green, J. M., & Murray, D. (1994). The use of the Edinburgh postnatal depression scale in research to explore the relationship between antenatal and postnatal dysphoria. In J. Cox & J. Holden (Eds.), *Perinatal psychiatry—Use and misuse of the Edinburgh Postnatal Depression Scale* (pp. 180-198). London: Gaskell.

Hayes, B. A., Muller, R., & Bradley, B. S. (2001). Perinatal depression: A randomised controlled trial of an antenatal education intervention for primiparas. *Birth, 28,* 28-35.

Hayes, B. A., Oriti, L., & Hingst, R. (1994). *Socio-demographic profile form.* Townsville, Australia: James Cook University, School of Nursing Sciences.

Hillier, C. A., & Slade, P. (1989). The impact of antenatal classes on knowledge, anxiety and confidence in primiparous women. *Journal of Reproductive Psychology, 7,* 3-13.

Kumar, R., & Robson, K. M. (1984). A prospective study of emotional disorders in childbearing women. *British Journal of Psychiatry, 144,* 35-47.

Lumley, J., & Austin, M. (2001). What interventions may reduce postnatal depression? *Current Opinion: Obstetrics and Gynecology, 13,* 605-611.

McNair, D. M., Lorr, M., & Droppleman, L. (1981). *Manual: Profile of mood states.* San Diego, CA: Education and Industrial Testing Service.

Meager, I., & Milgrom, J. (1996). Group treatment for postpartum depression: A pilot study. *Australian and New Zealand Journal of Psychiatry, 30,* 852-860.

Milgrom, J., Martin, P. R., & Negri, L. M. (1999). *Treating postnatal depression: A psychological approach for health care practitioners.* Chichester, UK: Wiley.

Norbeck, J. S. (1990). *Revised scoring instructions for the Norbeck Social Support Questionnaire.* San Francisco: School of Nursing, University of California.

Norbeck, J. S., Lindsey, A. M., & Carrieri, V. L. (1981). The development of an instrument to measure social support. *Nursing Research, 30,* 264-269.

O'Hara, M. W., Stuart, S., Gorman, L. L., & Wenzel, A. (2000). Efficacy of interpersonal psychotherapy for postpartum depression. *Archives of General Psychiatry, 57,* 1039-1045.

O'Hara, M. W., & Swain, A. M. (1996). Rates and risks of postnatal depression: A meta-analysis. *International Review of Psychiatry, 8,* 37-54.

O'Hara, M. W., Zekoski, E. M., & Philipps, L. H. (1990). Controlled prospective study of postpartum mood disorders: Comparison of childbearing and nonchildbearing women. *Journal of Abnormal Psychology, 99,* 3-15.

Pope, S., Watts, J., Evans, S., McDonald, S. J., & Henderson, J. (2000). *Postnatal depression: A systematic review of published scientific literature to 1999.* Canberra: Commonwealth of Australia (NHRMC).

Spitzer, R. L., Endicott, J., & Robins, E. (1981). *Research Diagnostic Criteria (RDC) for a selected group of functional disorders* (3rd ed.). New York: New York State Psychiatric Institute.

Stamp, G. E., Williams, A. S., & Crowther, C. A. (1995). Evaluation of antenatal and postnatal support to overcome postnatal depression: A randomised, controlled trial. *Birth, 22,* 138-143.

Wolkind, S., Coleman, E. Z., & Ghodisan, M. (1980). Continuities in maternal depression. *International Journal of Family Psychiatry, 1,* 167-181.

Acknowledgment. The study was supported by a grant from the National Health and Medical Research Council (No. 944134), Canberra, ACT, Australia.

5

Older Adults With Chronic Conditions: Reports on Depressive Symptoms

Jaclene A. Zauszniewski
Diana L. Morris
Sunida Preechawong
Hsiu-Ju Chang

Depression is the most common mental disorder among older adults in the United States (Blazer, 2003; Jeste et al., 1999; Sable, Dunn, & Zisook, 2002) and one of the most disabling conditions among older adults worldwide. In the US, more than 6 million adults age 65 and older, representing approximately 15% of older adults, suffer from clinical depression (Lavretsky, 2001; McCall, Parks, Smith, Pope, & Griggs, 2002; Sable et al., 2002). Prevalence estimates of depression in older adults range from about 5% in community samples to 20% in nursing home residents and nearly 30% of older adults seen in primary care settings (Alexopoulos, 2001; Brown, Lapane, & Luisi, 2002; Mulsant & Ganguli, 1999). About 50% of older adults who are hospitalized for medical illnesses, or are receiving long-term care, experience clinical depression (Alexopoulos, 2001; Koenig, Cohen, Blazer, Krishnan, & Sibert, 1993; Lebowitz, Pearson, & Schneider, 1997).

Older adults are particularly vulnerable to depression for a number of reasons, including chronic medical conditions, such as diabetes, stroke, heart disease, cancer, chronic lung disease, and arthritis (Bruce, 2002; Gottfries, 2001; Kraaij, Arensman, & Spinhoven, 2002; Oxman, Berkman, Kasl, Freeman, & Barrett, 1992; Sable et al., 2002). Approximately 80% of the elderly population has at least one of these chronic medical conditions (Fowles, 1994), any of which can trigger depression. In addition, older adults may experience limitations in their performance of daily activities of living, and these limitations are also associated with increased vulnerability to late-life depression (Husaini, 1997; Valderrama, Damian, Ruigomez, & Martin, 2002). In 2002, about 6 million older adults in the US needed assistance with daily activities (Husaini, 1997).

However, diagnosing depression in older adults is fraught with challenges (Alexopoulos, 2001; Garland & Solomons, 2002; Sable et al., 2002). Indeed, many studies have reported that in older adults, a depressed mood may not be as prominent as symptoms of irritability, anxiety, or physical or somatic symptoms and changes in functioning (Alexopoulos, 2001; Garland & Solomons, 2002; Sable et al., 2002). It is estimated that about 15% of older adults have depressive symptoms that do not meet the diagnostic criteria specified by the *Diagnostic and Statistical Manual* (4th ed.) for diagnosis of major depression (*DSM-IV*, American Psychiatric Association, 1994; Alexopoulos, 2001). Nevertheless, these older adults can experience depressive symptoms that lead to functional deficits in activities of daily living (ADL) and instrumental activities of daily living (IADL), compromising independence and quality of life (Lyness et al., 2002).

While depression is generally viewed as a clinical syndrome with specific diagnostic criteria, depression has also been conceptualized as a mood state or as a collection of symptoms (Beck, 1991). Because older adults may not meet specific diagnostic criteria for the clinical syndrome of depression, studies of older adults commonly use the term depression to mean depressive symptoms (Futterman, Thompson, Gallagher-Thompson, & Ferris, 1995). Depressed mood in older adults encompasses a range of affective responses (e.g., anxiety, irritability, etc.) that may differ from the predominantly depressed mood described in the diagnostic criteria for clinical depression (Futterman et al., 1995).

There is considerable disagreement in the literature about the effects of aging on depression (Jorm, 2000). For example, in a sample of healthy older adults (age 65 and older), Minicuci, Maggi, Pavan, Enzi, and Crepaldi (2002) reported no significant relationship between age and depressive symptoms. Yet Ehrlich and Isaacowitz (2002) found that older adults (age 60 and over) reported more depressive symptoms than middle-aged adults (ages 37 to 59). Similarly, Roberts, Kaplan, Shema, and Strawbridge (1997) reported that increasing age was associated with more depressive symptoms in community-dwelling adults 50 years and older. However, these researchers concluded that the apparent effects of aging on depressive symptoms were probably attributable to chronic health problems and functional impairments.

Older women are known to suffer more frequently from depressive symptoms than older men (Kockler & Heun, 2002; Minicuci et al., 2002; Sonnenberg, Beekman, Deeg, & van Tilburg, 2000), and the course and outcomes of late-life depression have been found to differ by gender (Lavretsky, 2002). However, the findings on gender differences in patterns of depressive symptoms in older adults are inconsistent. Forsell, Jorm, and Winblad (1994) reported that among community-dwelling older adults, depressed women displayed more mood-related symptoms while depressed men presented more motivational disturbances. Kockler and Heun (2002) found that while gender differences appeared to be more subtle in older adults than in younger populations, community-dwelling older women reported more appetite changes while older men described more feelings of agitation. Yet other studies found similar depressive symptom patterns among older men and women (Roberts, Kaplan, Shema, & Strawbridge, 1997; Sonnenberg et al., 2000). To date, no studies have examined whether there are gender differences in depressive symptoms or negative emotions among older adults with chronic conditions and functional limitations.

Older adults with chronic medical conditions commonly report symptoms that are often considered symptoms of clinical depression (Alexopoulos et al., 2002;

Blazer, 2003; Kurlowicz, 1997). However, a number of widely accepted and psychometrically sound measures of depression identify depressive symptoms that may in fact be symptoms of chronic illnesses, such as changes in sleep and activity patterns, appetite, and weight. Further, the currently available measures do not fully capture the range of emotional symptoms that may be associated with depressive illness in older adults.

This study therefore compared older adults' depressive symptoms collected from three measures:

1. the Center for Epidemiological Studies Depression (CES-D) Scale (Radloff, 1977);
2. the CES-D short form (Andresen, Malmgren, Carter, & Patrick, 1994); and
3. a new measure, the Emotional Symptom Checklist (ESC), which assesses negative emotions not captured by the standard instruments.

The study also examined the association of gender, age cohort, number of chronic conditions, and functional status with scores on the three measures. The study was part of a larger study that examined the effects of small group interventions on the psychosocial health of older adults with chronic conditions.

METHODS

Design and Sample. A descriptive, correlational design was used to examine depressive symptoms and negative emotions in older adults with chronic conditions, who resided in retirement communities (RCs) in northeast Ohio. RCs were defined as assisted living facilities and independent living facilities that provided services and assistance with daily activities for older adults. A sample of 314 residents who were willing to participate in the study was recruited from 29 RCs. To be included, residents had to be able to read, understand, and speak English; receive services or assistance with at least one of the basic or instrumental activities of daily living, including ambulation, toileting, meal preparation, shopping, and housework; and be cognitively intact as determined by a score of 7 or higher on the 10-item Short Portable Mental Status Questionnaire (SPMSQ; Pfeiffer, 1975).

Instruments. Demographic information was recorded to describe the sample. Age was recorded as the participant's reported age in years and birth date. Gender and race were recorded based on participant self-report.

The number and type of chronic conditions were measured using the questionnaire developed by Fillenbaum (1988) to assess the presence of chronic conditions (26 different disorders). This instrument provides a checklist for respondents to indicate whether or not they experience such conditions as arthritis, hypertension, diabetes, heart disease, and 22 other conditions. This is the same measure as the physical health component of the Older Adults Resources and Services (OARS) Multidimensional Functional Assessment Questionnaire (MFAQ; Fillenbaum, 1988).

Functional status was measured by the Health Assessment Questionnaire (HAQ; Fries, 1996). The HAQ includes 20 questions on the functioning of respondents during the past week. Functioning is assessed in eight component areas: dressing and grooming, arising, eating, walking, hygiene, reaching, gripping, and outdoor activities. Each component includes 2 to 3 questions. Responses are scored on a 4-point scale of ability ranging from "without any difficulty" to "unable to do." Scores for each of the eight components are added for a total score that ranges from 0 to 24. Lower scores indicate greater self-sufficiency in performing daily activities. This well-known measure has reported reliability and validity from over 500 studies of older adults (Bruce & Fries, 2003). Cronbach's alpha for this sample was .86.

Depressive symptoms were measured by the CES-D and the short form of the CES-D. The 20-item CES-D (Radloff, 1977) asks participants to rate the frequency with which they experienced each listed symptom during the week prior to the interview on a 4-point Likert-type scale ranging from "rarely" or "none of the time" (0), to "most" or "all of the time" (3). Scores range from 0 to 60; higher scores after reverse coding for 4 items indicate greater frequency of depressive symptoms. The scale is a widely reported valid measure, and it has been standardized for a variety of ages and racial groups. Alpha coefficients of .86 for frail elderly (Davidson, Feldman, & Crawford, 1994) and .82 for healthy older adults (Zauszniewski, 1997) have been reported. Cronbach's alpha for this sample was .85.

The short form of the CES-D contains 10 items from the original scale (Andresen et al., 1994). This 10-item scale was developed by a Research Group at Stanford University based on examination of correlations between the original 20 items and the total scale score. The short form eliminated items that appeared redundant; also, unlike the full version of the CES-D, this version does not contain items on changes in appetite. Andresen and colleagues found the shortened scale to be particularly useful in research with older adults, and it had acceptable reliability, with a test-retest coefficient of .71. Moreover, the shortened scale was significantly correlated with positive affect ($r = -.63$) and health status ($r = .37$). For this group of elderly, Cronbach's alpha was .76.

Negative emotions were measured by the ESC, developed by the investigators. The ESC assesses the presence of 10 negative emotions within the past 2 weeks that may reflect risk factors for depression in older adults and are not fully captured on standard measures of depressive symptoms: anxiousness, nervousness, tension, worry, anger, restlessness, irritability, sadness, loneliness, and unhappiness. For each symptom experienced, respondents receive 1 point; for those they do not experience, they receive a 0. Total scores can thus range from 0 to 10, with higher scores indicating more negative emotions. Cronbach's alpha was .76. Significant correlations between the ESC and the State Anxiety Inventory (STAI A-State; $r = .58, p < .001$) and the CES-D ($r = .59, p < .001$) in this sample provide evidence of construct validity.

Data Collection Procedures. Approval from the Institutional Review Board was obtained prior to data collection. Following informed consent, older adults were individually interviewed by trained data collectors in a private setting at a mutually agreed-upon time. During the initial interview, information on age, gender, race, and number and types of chronic conditions was obtained, and participants completed the CES-D and the ESC measures.

Data Analysis. Descriptive statistics, including measures of central tendency and dispersion, were used to compare scores on the three measures. Pearson's correlations among the measures were examined for direction and strength. Number and types of negative emotions reported by the older adults were examined using frequency distributions and descriptive statistics. Analysis of variance (ANOVA) was used to examine differences on the three measures by gender and by age cohort. Pearson's correlations were used to identify relationships between the three measures and number of chronic conditions and functional status.

RESULTS

About 80% (79.6%) of the sample were women ($n = 250$); 20.4% were men ($n = 64$). The majority of the older adults were Caucasian ($n = 291$); 22 were African American, and one was American Indian. Their ages ranged from 64 to 98 years, with a mean of 82.7 years. There were 43 older adults in the young-old age cohort (ages 64 through 74), 138 in the middle-old cohort (ages 75 through 84), and 133 in the old-old cohort (ages 85 and over). On average, the older adults reported three chronic conditions. The most common were arthritis (64.2%), high blood pressure (47.3%), heart trouble (35.5%), circulation problems (31.0%), and urinary tract disorders (26.0%). Less than 5% ($n = 14$) reported having no chronic conditions.

In this sample of 314 older adults, mean scores on the CES-D-20 ($M = 7.07$; $SD = 7.02$) and the CES-D-10 ($M = 4.54$; $SD = 4.34$) indicated that the older adults had few depressive symptoms. The correlation of the CES-D-10 mean score and the CES-D-20 mean score was statistically significant ($r = .94, p < .001$). Also, both forms of the CES-D were significantly correlated with the ESC ($r = .54, p < .001$). All three measures were significantly correlated in the expected direction with number of chronic conditions ($r = .24, p < .001$ for the CES-D-20, $r = .25, p < .001$ for the CES-D-10, and $r = .19, p < .001$ for the ESC) and functional status ($r = .28, p < .001$ for the CES-D-20, $r = .29, p < .001$ for the CES-D-10, and $r = .21, p < .001$ for the ESC).

Although the older women had higher mean scores on the long and short forms of the CES-D ($M = 7.24$; $SD = 6.92$; and $M = 4.64$; $SD = 4.26$, respectively) than the older men ($M = 6.45$; $SD = 7.41$; and $M = 4.16$; $SD = 4.67$, respectively), these differences were not significant. In an analysis by age cohort, no differences were found on the CES-D short or long forms. The correlation coefficients between the two CES-D measures and the ESC were somewhat stronger for the men ($r = .64, p < .001$ for the CES-D-20, and $r = .63, p < .001$ for the CES-D-10) than for the women ($r = .52$, for both; $p < .001$).

The young-old group of older adults had the lowest mean scores on both the long and short CES-D forms ($M = 5.28$; $SD = 6.45$; and $M = 3.65$, $SD = 4.29$, respectively). The middle-old group had a slightly higher mean score ($M = 7.38$; $SD = 7.44$)

than the old-old group ($M = 7.35$; $SD = 6.71$) on the CES-D long form, while the old-old group had a higher mean score ($M = 4.82$; $SD = 4.11$) than the middle-old group ($M = 4.54$; $SD = 4.57$) on the CES-D short form. Correlations between the CES-D short and long forms and the ESC were strongest in the young-old group ($r = .75$, $p < .001$ for the CES-D-10 and $r = .76$, $p < .001$ for the CES-D-20), followed by the middle-old group ($r = .52$ for both forms; $p < .001$ for the CES-D-20), and the old-old group ($r = .50$ for both forms; $p < .001$).

On the CES-D-20, using the standard cutoff of 16 or greater (Schein & Koenig, 1997), the percentage of older adults with depressive symptoms was 11.8% (n = 37), including 10.9% (n = 7) men and 12% (n = 30) women. Similarly, on the short form of CES-D, applying a cutoff of 10 or higher (Andresen et al., 1994), the percentage of those with depressive symptoms was 12.1% (n = 38), including 10.9% (n = 7) men and 12.4% (n = 31) women. The differences in the proportions of older adults above the standard cutoff scores on the two CES-D measures were also examined by age cohort. The percentage in the young-old group who exceeded the cutoff score indicative of severe depressive symptoms was lower (7% for both CES-D forms) than for the other two age cohorts. The highest percentage of older adults who exceeded the cutoff score was in the middle-old group (13.7%, long form; 15.2%, short form).

Although the mean scores on both forms of the CES-D suggested that these older adults had few depressive symptoms, the average number of negative emotions reported by the older adults was 2, with a range of 0 to 10. Approximately 68% of the older adults (n = 212) reported experiencing at least one negative emotion, including 62.5 % of the men (n = 40) and 68.8% of the women (n = 172). Analysis by age cohort revealed that 67.4% of the young-old (n = 29), 63.8% of the middle old (n = 50), and 71.4% of the old-old (n = 38) reported at least one negative emotion. About 35% of the total sample (n = 109) reported at least three negative emotions. Almost 10% (n = 31) reported six or more negative emotions. Table 5.1 shows the number, frequency, and percent of older adults reporting their experience of the ten negative emotions.

In the total sample, sadness was the most commonly reported negative emotion (29%), followed by loneliness (28.7%), nervousness (26.4%), worry (24.5%), and anxiousness (23.9%). However, men reported loneliness (25%) and irritability (21.9%) most frequently, while women were more likely to report sadness (31.2%) and loneliness (29.6%). Both the young-old and middle-old adults reported sadness most frequently (25.6% and 33.3%, respectively); the middle-old also reported nervousness (33.3%). The old-old age cohort reported loneliness (30.8%) most frequently.

To further examine the relationships between negative emotions (ESC) and depressive symptoms measured by the CES-D-20 and the CES-D-10, participants were divided into three groups:

1. those with no negative emotions (n = 102);
2. those experiencing one or two negative emotions (n = 103); and
3. those experiencing at least three negative emotions (n = 109).

Using analysis of variance (ANOVA), the results indicated that the mean scores on the CES-D-10 and the CES-D-20 for older adults who reported experiencing at least three negative emotions ($M = 7.58$; $SD = 4.96$, and $M = 11.90$; $SD = 8.17$) were significantly higher than for those who reported experiencing less than three negative emotions ($M = 3.52$; $SD = 2.98$, and $M = 5.70$; $SD = 4.91$; $p < .001$). However, in this group of older adults, mean scores failed to meet the cutoff criterion of 16 on the CES-D-20 or 10 on the CES-D-10.

DISCUSSION

Several instruments are available for measuring the presence and severity of depressive symptoms in adults (Norris & Woehr, 1998). However, depressed older adults are more likely to express somatic complaints and less likely to report affective symptoms than younger adults (Kim, Pilkonis, Frank, Thase, & Reynolds, 2002). Valid measurement of depressive symptoms is further complicated by the fact that

TABLE 5.1. Number, Frequency, and Percent of Negative Emotions Reported by Older Adults

Number of Emotions	Total Sample (n = 314)	Female (n = 250)	Male (n = 64)	Young-Old (n = 43)	Middle-Old (n = 138)	Old-Old (n = 133)
None	102.0 (32.5%)	78.0 (31.2%)	24.0 (37.5%)	14.0 (32.6%)	50.0 (36.2%)	38.0 (28.6%)
One	62.0 (19.7%)	48.0 (19.2%)	14.0 (21.9%)	10.0 (23.3%)	23.0 (16.7%)	29.0 (21.8%)
Two	41.0 (13.1%)	32.0 (12.8%)	9.0 (14.1%)	7.0 (16.3%)	14.0 (10.1%)	20.0 (15.0%)
Three	35.0 (11.1%)	29.0 (11.6%)	6.0 (9.4%)	3.0 (7.0%)	15.0 (10.9%)	17.0 (12.8%)
Four	27.0 (8.6%)	22.0 (8.8%)	5.0 (7.8%)	4.0 (9.3%)	11.0 (8.0%)	12.0 (9.0%)
Five	16.0 (5.1%)	14.0 (5.6%)	2.0 (3.1%)	1.0 (2.3%)	10.0 (7.2%)	5.0 (3.8%)
Six	15.0 (4.8%)	14.0 (5.6%)	1.0 (1.6%)	1.0 (2.3%)	8.0 (5.8%)	6.0 (4.5%)
Seven	6.0 (1.9%)	5.0 (2.0%)	1.0 (1.6%)	2.0 (4.7%)	2.0 (1.4%)	2.0 (1.5%)
Eight	5.0 (1.6%)	4.0 (1.6%)	1.0 (1.6%)	— —	4.0 (2.9%)	1.0 (0.8%)
Nine	4.0 (1.3%)	3.0 (1.2%)	1.0 (1.6%)	1.0 (2.3%)	1.0 (0.7%)	2.0 (1.5%)
Ten	1.0 (0.3%)	1.0 (0.4%)	— —	— —	— —	1.0 (0.8%)

many older adults experience chronic conditions with symptoms that are similar to the symptoms of depression (Schein & Koenig, 1997; Turvey, Wallace, & Herzog, 1999). Thus, it is essential to find measures that accurately capture older adults' depressive symptoms. In addition, measures are needed that do not tax the energy of older adults, particularly those who live with chronic illness (Irwin, Artin, & Oxman, 1999).

In this study, scores on the CES-D-10 scale were highly correlated with those on the 20-item CES-D scale, supporting the use of the shorter scale with chronically ill older adults. These findings from older adults with chronic conditions and functional limitations are consistent with those of Andresen and colleagues (1994), who tested the short form of the CES-D with healthy older adults. Only 12% of the older adults in this study had CES-D scores that met the cutoff for a significant level of depressive symptoms. However, approximately 68% (n = 212) of the older adults reported having at least one negative emotion that may be a risk factor for or associated with depression. Thirty-three percent reported experiencing two to four negative emotions and 15% reported five or more negative emotions. The two most frequently reported negative emotions were sadness and loneliness, which may reflect a depressed mood. Depressed mood is the essential feature of depressive disorders (*DSM-IV*, American Psychiatric Association, 1994) but it has not been found to be prominent in older adults (Alexopoulos, 2001; Garland & Solomons, 2002; Sable et al., 2002).

The lack of significant gender differences in depressive symptoms in this sample of older adults with chronic conditions is consistent with the studies of community samples of healthy older adults conducted by Roberts and colleagues (1997) and Sonnenberg and associates (2000). The analysis by age cohort revealed a trend toward increasing depressive symptoms with age; though the differences between groups were not significant, this may reflect the unequal group sizes.

A majority of these older adults were willing to report the negative emotions they experienced. It may be that the format and context in which the questions were presented made them more comfortable in sharing such information than they might be in a clinical encounter. It may be easier to respond to simple yes-no items asking about the presence of specific emotions than to respond to detailed items with a number of response options. The measures were completed during an interview at their place of residence at a place and time convenient to them.

The older adults' negative emotion scores were strongly correlated with both CES-D scales. The use of the CES-D with the ESC, which obtains data specific on negative emotions, may be helpful in distinguishing between symptoms of major depression and those of subsyndromal or minor depression. The question is how to determine what number and severity of depressive symptoms and which negative emotions are indicators of minor depression in older adults. Currently there are no clear diagnostic criteria for this syndrome. The *DSM-IV* suggests that minor depression exists when one to two symptoms are present for 2 weeks, and in this study, 33% of the participants reported one or two negative emotions for that time frame. Recently, however, Williams and associates (2000) adapted the criteria to three to four symptoms for 4 weeks. Although 20% of the older adults in this study reported three or four negative emotions over 2 weeks, we do not know how long these feelings persisted and whether or not these persons would meet the proposed criteria for subsyndromal or minor depression. This is a significant issue for geriatric health care since even subsyndromal symptoms can interfere with older adults' ability to function in daily activities and quality of life and may be risk factors for major depression.

Older adults with chronic illnesses receive the majority of their care from primary health care providers (Unutzer, 2002), who are the front line in identifying mental health problems in older adults. The ESC could be used by clinicians to help older clients share information about the emotions they are experiencing and screen for depressive emotions. Although not diagnostic, high scores on the ESC suggest the presence of emotional symptoms not assessed by the CES-D and the need for additional screening for depression. The 10-item short form CES-D, an efficient and reliable screening tool, could then be used as part of a clinical assessment to determine the possible presence of clinical depression (Andresen et al., 1994). Scores below the cutoff for major depression could be used to identify clients at risk or experiencing minor depression.

REFERENCES

Alexopoulos, G. S. (2001). Interventions for depressed elderly primary care patients. *International Journal of Geriatric Psychiatry, 16*(6), 553-559.

Alexopoulos, G. S., Borson, S., Cuthbert, B. N., Devanand, D. P., Mulsant, B. H., Olin, J. T., & Oslin, D. W. (2002). Assessment of late life depression. *Biological Psychiatry, 52,* 164-174.

American Psychiatric Association. (1994). *Diagnosis and statistical manual of mental disorders* (4th ed.). Washington, DC: Author.

Andresen, E. M., Malmgren, J. A., Carter, W. B., & Patrick, D. L. (1994). Screening for depression in well older adults: Evaluation of a short form of the CES-D. *American Journal of Preventive Medicine, 10*(2), 77-84.

Blazer, D. G. (2003). Depression in late life: Review and commentary. *Journals of Gerontology: Series A: Biological Science & Medical Science, 58A*(3), 249-265.

Beck, A. T. (1991). Cognitive therapy as the integrative therapy. *Journal of Psychotherapy Integration, 1*(3), 191-198.

Brown, M. N., Lapane, K. L., & Luisi, A. F. (2002). The management of depression in older nursing home residents. *Journal of the American Geriatrics Society, 50*(1), 69-76.

Bruce, M. L. (2002). Psychosocial risk factors for depressive disorders in late life. *Biological Psychiatry, 52*(3), 175-184.

Bruce, M., & Fries, J. (2003). The Stanford Health Assessment Questionnaire: A review of its history, issues, progress, and documentation. *The Journal of Rheumatology, 30*(1), 167-178.

Davidson, H., Feldman, P. H., & Crawford, S. (1994). Measuring depressive symptoms in the frail elderly. *Journals of Gerontology, 49*(4), 159-164.

Ehrlich, B. S., & Isaacowitz, D. M. (2002). Does subjective well-being increase with age? *Perspectives in Psychology, 5,* 20-26.

Fillenbaum, G. G. (1988). *Multidimensional functional assessment of older adults: The Duke Older Americans Resources and Services Procedures.* Hillsdale, NJ: Erbaum.

Forsell, Y., Jorm, A. F., & Winblad, B. (1994). Association of age, sex, cognitive dysfunction, and disability with major depressive symptoms in an elderly sample. *The American Journal of Psychiatry, 151*(11), 1600-1604.

Fowles, D. (1994). *A profile of older Americans.* Washington, DC: American Association of Retired Persons.

Fries, J. F. (1996). The Health Assessment Questionnaire. In I. McDowell & C. Newell (Eds.), *Measuring health: A guide to rating scales and questionnaires* (2nd ed., pp. 106-115). New York: Oxford University Press.

Futterman, A., Thompson, L. W., Gallagher-Thompson, D., & Ferris, R. (1995). Depression in later life: Epidemiology, assessment, etiology, and treatment. In E. E. Beckham (Ed.), *Handbook of Depression* (pp. 494-538). New York: The Guilford Press.

Garland, E. J., & Solomons, K. (2002). Early detection of depression in young and elderly people. *British Columbia Medical Journal, 44*(9), 469-472.

Gottfries, C. G. (2001). Late life depression. *European Archives of Psychiatry & Clinical Neuroscience, 251*(Suppl. 2), 57-61.

Husaini, B. A. (1997). Predictors of depression among the elderly: Racial differences over time. *American Journal of Orthopsychiatry, 67*(1), 48-58.

Irwin, M., Artin, K. H., & Oxman, M. N. (1999). Screening for depression in the older adult: Criterion validity of the 10-item Center for Epidemiological Studies Depression Scale (CES-D). *Archives of Internal Medicine, 159*(15), 1701-1704.

Jeste, D. V., Alexopoulos, G. S., Bartels, S. J., Cummings, J. L., Gallo, J. J., Gottlieb, G. L., Halpain, M. C., Palmer, B. W., Patterson, T. L., Reynolds, C. F., & Lebowitz, B. D. (1999). Consensus statement on the upcoming crisis in geriatric mental health: Research agenda for the next 2 decades. *Archives of General Psychiatry, 56*(9), 848-853.

Jorm, A. F. (2000). Does old age reduce the risk of anxiety and depression? A review of epidemiological studies across the adult life span. *Psychological Medicine, 30*(1), 11-22.

Kim, Y., Pilkonis, P. A., Frank, A., Thase, M. E., & Reynolds, C. F. (2002). Differential functioning of the Beck Depression Inventory in late-life patients: Use of item response theory. *Psychology and Aging, 17*(3), 379-391.

Kockler, M., & Heun, R. (2002). Gender differences of depressive symptoms in depressed and nondepressed elderly persons. *International Journal of Geriatric Psychiatry, 17,* 65-72.

Koenig, H. G., Cohen, H. J., Blazer, D. G., Krishnan, K. R., & Sibert, T. E. (1993). Profile of depressive symptoms in younger and older medical inpatients with major depression. *Journal of the American Geriatrics Society, 41*(11), 1169-1176.

Kraaij, V., Arensman, E., & Spinhoven, P. (2002). Negative life events and depression in elderly persons: A meta-analysis. *The Journals of Gerontology Series B: Psychological Sciences and Social Sciences, 57,* 87-94.

Kurlowicz, L. H. (1997). Barriers to recognition of depression in hospitalized older adults. *Image: Journal of Nursing Scholarship, 29*(1), 96.

Lavretsky, H. (2001). Choosing appropriate treatment for geriatric depression. *Clinical Geriatrics, 9*(5), 30-46.

Lebowitz, B. D., Pearson, J. L., & Schneider, L. S. (1997). Diagnosis and treatment of depression in late life: Consensus statement update. *Journal of the American Medical Association, 278*(16), 1186-1190.

Lyness, J. M., Caine, E. D., King, D. A., Conwell, Y., Duberstein, P. R., & Cox, C. (2002). Depressive disorders and symptoms in older primary care patients: One-year outcomes. *American Journal of Geriatric Psychiatry, 10*(3), 275-282.

McCall, N. T., Parks, P., Smith, K., Pope, G., & Griggs, M. (2002). The prevalence of major depression or dysthymia among aged Medicare Fee-for-Service beneficiaries. *International Journal of Geriatric Psychiatry, 17*(6), 557-565.

Minicuci, N., Maggi, S., Pavan, M., Enzi, G., & Crepaldi, G. (2002). Prevalence rate and correlates of depressive symptoms in older individuals: The Veneto Study. *Journal of Gerontology: Series A, 57A*(3), M155-M161.

Mulsant, B. H., & Ganguli, M. (1999). Epidemiology and diagnosis of depression in late life. *Journal of Clinical Psychiatry, 60*(Suppl. 20), 9-15.

Norris, M. P., & Woehr, M. D. (1998). Differentiating somatic symptoms in the elderly: Depression, aging, or illness? *Journal of Mental Health and Aging, 4*(3), 347-359.

Oxman, T. E., Berkman, L. F., Kasl, S., Freeman, D. H., Jr., & Barrett, J. (1992). Social support and depressive symptoms in the elderly. *American Journal of Epidemiology, 135*(4), 356-368.

Pfeiffer, E. (1975). A short portable mental status questionnaire for the assessment of organic brain deficit in elderly patients. *Journal of the American Geriatrics Society, 23,* 433-441.

Radloff, L. S. (1977). The CES-D scale: A self-report depression scale for research in the general population. *Applied Psychological Measurement, 1,* 385-401.

Roberts, R. E., Kaplan, G. A., Shema, S. J., & Strawbridge, W. J. (1997). Prevalence and correlates of depression in an aging cohort: The Alameda County study. *Journal of Gerontology: Series B, 52*(5), S252-258.

Sable, J. A., Dunn, L. B., & Zisook, S. (2002). Late-life depression: How to identify its symptoms and provide effective treatment. *Geriatrics, 57*(2),18-19, 22-23, 26.

Schein, R. L., & Koenig, H. G. (1997). The Center for Epidemiological Studies-Depression (CES-D) Scale: Assessment of depression in the medically ill elderly. *International Journal of Geriatric Psychiatry, 12*(4), 436-446.

Sonnenberg, C. M., Beekman, A. T. F., Deeg, D. J. H., & van Tilburg, W. (2000). Sex difference in late-life depression. *Acta Psychiatrica Scandinavica, 101*(4), 286-292.

Turvey, C. L., Wallace, R. B., & Herzog, R. (1999). A revised CES-D measure of depressive symptoms and a DSM-based measure of major depressive episodes in the elderly. *International Psychogeriatrics, 11*(2), 139-148.

Unutzer, J. (2002). Diagnosis and treatment of older adults with depression in primary care. *Biological Psychiatry, 52*(3), 285-292.

Valderrama, G. E., Damian, J., Ruigomez, A., & Martin, M. J. (2002). Chronic disease, functional status, and self-ascribed causes of disabilities among noninstitutionalized older people Spain. *Journal of Gerontology: Series A, 57A*(11), M716-M721.

Williams, J. W., Jr,, Barrett, J., Oxman, T., Frank, E., Katon, W., & Sullivan, M. (2000). Treatment of dysthymia and minor depression in primary care: A randomized controlled trial in older adults. *Journal of the American Medical Association, 284*(12), 1519-1526.

Zauszniewski, J. A. (1997). Evaluation of a measure of learned resourcefulness for elders. *Journal of Nursing Measurement, 5,* 71-86.

Acknowledgment. Data taken from a larger study funded by National Institute for Nursing Research, National Institutes of Health (R01-04428). The authors acknowledge the editorial assistance of Elizabeth M. Tornquist of the University of North Carolina at Chapel Hill.

6

The Impact of War Stress on the Health of Lebanese Families

Laila F. Farhood

Family stress research has received increased attention in the last decade. Family researchers have struggled with the issue of developing theories aimed at uncovering why some families are better able to cope with life stress, while other families are exhausted and succumb in the face of hardships. McCubbin and McCubbin (1987) and Olson and McCubbin (1989) introduced the notion of family types and expanded on family resources such as coping and appraisal. This conceptualization attempts to guide researchers in identifying family types, strengths, and capabilities which are often called upon to manage a major transition and change which is needed for family reorganization and adaptation.

Most research concerned with stressful life events and their effect on mental health has been conducted in the West and relates to nonwar situations and to individuals rather than families. Research dealing with health effects of crisis situations is limited either to natural disasters or to combat situations. War-related studies eliciting the impact on the civilian population are mostly descriptive and exploratory in nature and point to a need for further research which takes into consideration the experience and perception of individual family members, as well as the family as a unit. Moreover, families are subjected to different levels of stress with a varied intensity and perception. A major question relates to the quality of health outcome in families subjected to high and low levels of stress and to the resources needed to safeguard the family against the impact of stress. The issue gets even more entangled in a war situation where families are subjected to the intense war stress in addition to the nonwar transitional life events.

The war in Lebanon (1975-1991) began with seemingly unrelated incidents that led to bouts of fighting between political factions. Violent rounds in the capital intensified in magnitude to include street fighting, random explosions, kidnapping, and torture, as well as cross-shelling of residential areas with rockets and field artillery (Sha'ar & Bryce, 1986). A demarcation green line divided the capital, Beirut, into two sectors, East and West, cutting family and friends from their support systems. In addition, the commercial center of the city was destroyed; the seaport and major banks were vandalized and looted by different warring factions.

The airport was closed, the seaport was taken over by one major militia, the power plants were bombed, and consequently electricity and water supplies were cut off for several months. The impact of war on the Lebanese family was traumatic and manifested itself in psychological, physical, depressive, and interpersonal symptoms. The mediating role of social support and resources was also reported (Farhood et al., 1993).

This chapter aims at predicting family adaptation outcomes in high and low perceived stress groups for war and nonwar events. It will identify a set of predictors that discriminates between high and low stress experienced by families.

A growing body of literature shows that persons exposed to acts of war suffer differentially from a set of problems as a result of such acts. However, the impact on the family seems to be more complex. In her study, Farhood (1999) tested a model predicting family adaptation. Results revealed that perceived stress, social support, and family resources were important predictors of family adaptation. Family adaptation was measured by the family's physical and mental health.

The impact of war conditions on health status seems to occur because experiencing war produces a variety of stressful life experiences, as well as a wide range of psychiatric disorders like depression, anxiety and poor interpersonal relations (Kaplan, Roberts, Camacho, & Coyne, 1987; McCubbin, Joy, Couble, Patterson, & Needle, 1980; Schlenger, Caddely, & Elbert, 2002). In Lebanon, studies have examined the health consequences of the war. Farhood and colleagues (1993), and Karam and Bou Ghosn (2003) studied the impact of war stress among family and individual members who have been subjected to a traumatic and continuous process of war stress for 16 years. Findings suggest that war stress causes significant impact on the physical and mental health of the family members, namely mothers, fathers, and adolescents. The authors also reported the role of mediating factors such as a social support system in alleviating the intensity and impact of war stress. In another study, Farhood (1999) tested a model of family stress and adaptation among Lebanese families. Findings revealed that perceived war stress and social support were consistent predictors of family adaptation.

Life events literature also speaks of the role of high stress and changes in the family system. Holmes and Masuda (1974) reported that there is considerable evidence that links the accumulation of life events to onset of illness: The greater the magnitude of life events, the greater the risk of illness, and furthermore, the greater the seriousness of the chronic illness. Magnitude estimates or rated perceptions of life event severity and the frequency of occurrence of life event vary. People of differing characteristics and cultures not only perceive the significance of life events differently, but also report a difference in the quality and quantity of life events occurrence (Garrity & Marx, 1985; Holmes & Masuda, 1974; Zegans, 1982).

Zegans (1982) reported that people react to life situations in terms of the meaning of those situations to them. The greater the magnitude of such life events and the more stressful they are perceived to be, the greater the risk of acquiring an illness of a serious nature (Holmes & Masuda, 1974; Holmes & Rahe, 1967). Patterns of disruptive impact of life events assume that certain events require more intense and prolonged coping efforts than do others. The greater the strain on the coping mechanisms, the more likely that inadequate or inappropriate responses will be utilized, thus eliciting idiosyncratic or pathological physiological reactions.

Although this study does not test posttraumatic stress disorder (PTSD) in families, the literature supports the importance of the level of exposure and symptomatology. For example, symptoms of PTSD following natural disasters and war situations increased with the level of exposure and presence of other stressful life events (Farhood & Noureddine, 2003; Green, 1994; Hardin, Weinrich, Weinrich, Hardin, & Garrison, 1994). Also, the degree of exposure was found to positively correlate with PTSD severity 1 1/2 years after the 1988 earthquake in Armenia (Goenjian et al., 1994).

The relationship between life events and illness outcomes has been established. However, other dimensions of life events are also important: intensity versus mildness, perception and control over those events, influence and characterize the response of the family (Lipman-Blumen, 1975; Pearlin, Liberman, Menaghan, Mullan, 1981; Rotter, 1966; Zegans, 1982). Burr (1973) cited the influence of variables such as the severity of the event and the intensity of exposure, and the family's definition of the situation. Also, previous exposure to other traumatic events and losses following the disaster were important predictors in the response (Garrison et al., 1995). An association was found between high stress and low functioning in subjects with psychiatric disorders (Persson, Runeson & Wasserman, 1999). Moreover, Hill (1949, 1958) defined crisis-prone families as those experiencing more frequent and severe stressful life events, who define more of these events as crises than non-crisis-prone families.

It is believed that the Lebanese civil war is unique in providing rich research material about war-related stressful life events. The majority of the population was affected and exposed, with minimal individual or family control over events. However, families differ in their reaction to such happenings and in their handling of such situations; this makes them different in outcome characteristics. It is therefore logical to assume that reactions to war stress are affected both by characteristics of the stressful situations such as intensity and perception and by individual family characteristics. Even for the first category, research has shown that subjective perception of life events is more important than their objective nature (Farhood, 1999; Farhood et al., 1993; McCubbin et al., 1980). Also, traumatic life events and high stress were predictors of physical and psychological distress among Lebanese prisoners of war (Saab, Chaaya, Doumit, & Farhood, 2003) and of PTSD, depression, and health status in Lebanese civilians exposed to a church explosion (Farhood & Noureddine, 2003).

The aim of this study was to compare high- and low-stress Lebanese families on the basis of their perceived life events with respect to war and nonwar stressors, and to identify a set of predictors (family adaptation) that can discriminate between high- and low-stress families. It is believed that low-stress families will indicate more positive family adaptation, reflected by their physical health, psychological health, depression, and interpersonal and marital relationships.

The theoretical framework for this study is grounded in family stress theory based on the model tested and presented in an earlier study (Farhood, 1999). The model included three main sets of concepts:

1. stressors and perceived stress, particularly those generated by the war experience;
2. family resources that intervene to protect against these factors; and
3. health outcomes for the family.

Figure 6.1 portrays the direct and indirect linkages among model variables and the expected relationships between them which was examined in an earlier study (Farhood, 1999). In testing the model, multiple regression analyses revealed that it was perceived stress, rather than the objective occurrence of events, that predicted family adaptation. However, the more objective events experienced, the greater their perception as stressful, which led, in turn, to less positive family adaptation. Family resources, particularly social support, directly and positively impacted family adaptation, and were also associated with increased use of cognitive coping. In addition, social support and education were predictors of physical health and depression, while social support and economic status were predictors of interpersonal relationships. Cognitive coping did not predict either health or interactional outcomes but was associated with higher levels of social support, education, and economic status (Farhood, 1999).

In this study families were classified into high and low stress for the purpose of predicting family adaptation outcome, based on their level of perceived war and nonwar stress. The objective stressors encompass both war-related stressors, to which families were exposed because of the war situation in Lebanon, and nonwar-related stressors that were experienced by families irrespective of their war-related experiences. The model included the family's perceived stress. While presumed to be related strongly, perceptions do not necessarily correlate completely with objective experience (Farhood, 1999). In this study perceived stress was used and defined as the subjective perception of war and nonwar stressors experienced, measured in terms of perceived impact of each life event.

Health was conceptualized to include physical and mental health and interactional outcomes such as interpersonal and marital relationships. Family adaptation encompasses both health and interactional outcomes. Health outcomes include both the physical and the psychological dimensions of health which are sensitive to stress. Included are physical symptoms that individuals may experience in the form of somatization, as well as psychological symptoms associated with depression and with other forms of mental illness. Interactional outcomes include problems in interpersonal and marital relations.

Family was defined as a unit of members living together and related by kinship. For purposes of this study the family included at least two and a maximum of three members; the mother, father, and one adolescent child chosen at random.

The study hypothesis stated that when high- and low-stress families are compared on the basis of their perceived life events score for war and nonwar stress and a combination of the two, the low-stress groups will indicate more positive

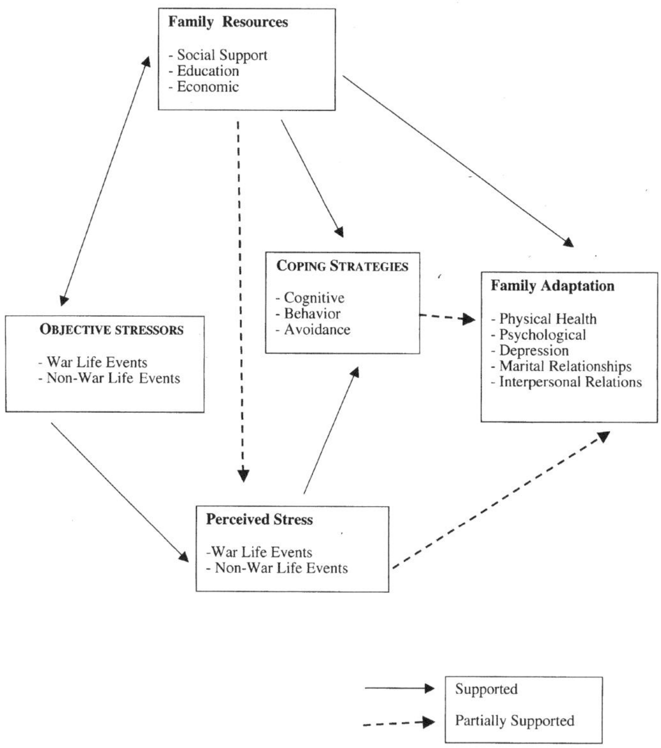

Figure 6.1. Model predicting family adaptation.

family adaptation as reflected by physical health, psychological health, depression, and interpersonal and marital relationships.

METHODS

SAMPLE

The sample for the study comprised 540 families. From each block in West Beirut included in the Beirut Health survey (Zurayk & Armenian, 1985), a proportional random sample was drawn from the families. From this group of families, 438 met the study criteria and were included in the study. Each family had at least two persons and a maximum of three persons in the family: the mother, father, and an adolescent chosen at random from among his/her siblings. The sample consisted of 188 families with mothers, fathers, and an adolescent; 217 families with mothers and fathers; and 33 families with mothers and adolescents (438 mothers, 405 fathers, and 221 adolescents). The average age of the parents was 46.7; the majority were married.

INSTRUMENTS

The instruments were designed by a team of investigators at the American University of Beirut and were written in Arabic. Measures were modifications of previously devised instruments validated on the Lebanese population (Farhood et al., 1993), and measured the main aspects of family adaptation (physical and psychological health, depression, and interpersonal and marital relationships), war and nonwar life events as stressors (frequency of occurrence and perception of stress). Measures were derived from scales that had been used on the Lebanese population (Bryce, Walker, Ghorayeb, & Kanj, 1989; Farhood et al., 1993). The reliability and validity of the measures were ascertained through pilot testing, assessing content validity, and computing internal consistency reliability of the scales. Cronbach's alpha was equal or greater than 0.70 for each of the scales (α for depression = 0.77, psychological = 0.73, physical = 0.73, marital = 0.71, interpersonal = 0.71). The scales were further subjected to content validation. Respondents were asked to rate severity of symptoms on a 4-point scale.

The instruments consisted of the following questionnaires:

1. A health symptoms questionnaire for adults which covered every individual 12 years of age or older, each responding for himself/herself. Information comprised current complaints of physical symptoms, psychological symptoms, depression, and interpersonal and marital relationships.
2. A life events questionnaire which gathered information from the mother, father and an adolescent chosen at random from among the adolescents in the family. The questionnaire included war- and nonwar-related life events that the family had been exposed to in the recent past, with an evaluation of the perception and seriousness of impact. Mothers', fathers', and adolescents' reporting of those events correlated. The mother's ratings were thus used as the family war-events score.

MEASUREMENT OF CONCEPTS AND INSTRUMENTS

A family score was computed by averaging the scores of individual family members on that variable rated on a 4-point scale according to frequency of occurrence, with a summative score. Reporting was restricted to 6 months prior to the interview. A summary score was obtained for each individual by adding the severity elements for the symptoms. A family score on depression, psychological, physical, marital, and interpersonal measures was obtained by averaging individual family scores for each family (Feetham, 1991).

Physical Health. Somatization reflecting physical response to stress and measured by obtaining information on 14 somatic complaints adapted from the *Diagnostic and Statistical Manual of Mental Disorders* (DSM-IV; American Psychiatric Association, 2000). Physical symptoms included headache, faintness and dizziness, pain in the chest, muscle pain, low back or neck pain, constipation, diarrhea, nausea, vomiting, shortness of breath, pharyngitis, running nose, allergic reactions, and eye strain.

Mental Health. This dimension addresses both depression as well as psychological symptoms.

1. Depression was assessed by obtaining information on 16 symptoms, based on the Beck Depression Inventory (Beck & Steer, 1993; DSM-IV, 2000). The symptoms included change in sleep patterns, appetite, and weight; loss of interest and pleasure; blaming self; crying easily; inability to concentrate; fatigue; and suicidal thoughts.
2. Psychological symptoms other than depression were assessed by obtaining information on seven commonly used complaints (DSM- IV, 2000) such as nervousness, tremors, trembling, heart pounding, feeling fearful, sudden scares, avoidance of activities and places, and forgetfulness.

Interactional Outcomes. These comprise interpersonal and marital relations.

1. Interpersonal relationships were assessed by asking about six problem areas that could arise in relating to others. The degree of change from before the war was queried for each problem. The problem areas included quick anger with difficulty in control, being argumentative and quarrelsome, difficulty in maintaining social relations, isolating oneself, and feelings that others do not understand him/her.
2. Marital relations were examined in terms of problems or difficulties that a couple may experience. These areas included misunderstanding, being argumentative, conflict about male and female role expectations, social issues, religious issues, sexual issues, child rearing, in-laws, and financial issues.

War and Nonwar Stressors. These were addressed as follows:

1. War-related events consisted of 17 events possibly experienced by family such as displacement, armed combat in residential area, kidnapping of family member, injury, death, damage to house, and events related to daily hassles such as cuts in electricity, water shortage, crossing the green line separating East and West Beirut, inability to visit family and friends, and events associated with deterioration of the economic situation and inability to meet the basic necessities due to the war. Respondents were asked if they experienced any of these events during the past 6 months, and in the past 2 years for very serious events such as kidnapping or killing of family members/or friends. The score was the total number of affirmative responses.
2. Nonwar-related events comprised 18 stressful life events during the last 6 months associated with natural events such as: birth; pregnancy; abortion; divorce; marriage or death in the family; immigration of a family member; relative; or a close friend; troubles at work for a family member; loss of a job, wife starting work; retirement; and serious problem facing a family member, relative, or friend. A summative score was derived in a similar fashion to war-related events.

Because of the consistency of mothers', fathers', and adolescents' reporting on war and nonwar events, the mothers' ratings were used as the family war and nonwar events scores.

Perceived Stress. This was defined as the subjective perception of war and nonwar stressors experienced, measured in terms of the perceived impact of each life event on a 4-point scale with 0 for the event not occurring or having no impact, 1 for mild, 2 for moderate, and 3 for severe impact. A summative score was obtained by adding the impact element for each family in the study across the events. Each family, then, had one family score for war and nonwar events and for other study variables.

PROCEDURES

Families were interviewed at their Beirut residences by trained university graduate students who were fluent in both Arabic and English. Written informed consent was obtained. Participation in the study was voluntary and involved no personal risk. Confidentiality and anonymity were assured. The study was approved by the university human subjects protection committee. The field work started after an intensive period of training. The interviewing was undertaken by a group of 25 students and graduates from the American University of Beirut. The interviewers were supervised by four research assistants and the principal investigator.

DATA ANALYSIS

Discriminant analysis was employed to differentiate high- and low-stress families with respect to physical health, psychological health, depression, and interpersonal and marital relationships. The major purpose of discriminant function analysis was to describe major differences among the high and low groups and to provide prediction about membership in high and low stress categories. Stepwise variable selection, a hierarchal approach, was also used. Moreover, canonical discriminant function also checked for the overall significance. These techniques helped identify to what extent do families who demonstrated extreme levels of (a) perceived war stress, (b) perceived nonwar stress, and (c) a combination of the two, differ in physical and mental health, and marital and interpersonal relationships. A significant difference between groups implies that, given a set of scores, one can predict which group that set comes from. The probability value was set at 0.05 level.

Families were classified into low- and high-stress groups based on their score for perceived war and nonwar life events and a combination of the two. For war stress, families with scores ranging from zero to 8.9 fell into the low-stress category ($Mdn = 9.0$), and families with a score of 9 or higher fell into the high-stress category. A median split ($Mdn = 3.5$) was also applied for the nonwar stress. Those with scores of zero to 3.5 constituted the low-stress, and those with scores of 3.51 or higher, the high-stress groups. Cross-tabulation of these two groups yielded four groups as shown in Table 6.1.

RESULTS

Table 6.2 presents a summary of family responses on the study variables as an average summative score computed for each family based on the number of individu-

TABLE 6.1. Cross Classification of Perceived War and Perceived Nonwar Groups

	Nonwar Stress		
War Stress	Low	High	Total
Low	138	80	218 (49.8%)
High	83	137	220 (50.2%)
Total	221 (50.5%)	217 (49.5%)	438 (100.0%)

TABLE 6.2. Distribution of Family Variables Families in Sample (*N* = 438)

Variable	Range	*M*	*SD*	*Mdn*
Average Age	21.0-80.5	46.7	11.35	45.5
Objective Stress				
War Events	0.0-14.0	5.6	2.36	5.0
Nonwar	1.0-11.0	2.9	1.65	3.0
Perceived Stress				
War Stress	0.0-24.5	9.4	4.45	9.0
Nonwar	1.0-19.0	4.2	2.8	3.5
Physical	0.0-29.0	6.5	5.42	5.0
Psychological	0.0-21.0	5.1	4.11	4.0
Depression	10.4-48.0	22.99	6.55	21.0
Interpersonal	7.0-33.0	16.99	4.89	17.0
Marital	0.0-17.5	3.4	3.61	2.5

als in the family unit. The maximum score for each scale was composed of the number of items multiplied by the severity impact. Evaluation of assumptions of linearity, normality, multicollinearity, and homogeneity of variance-covariance matrices revealed no threat to multivariate analysis.

Except for slightly skewed distribution, the values, for skewness and kurtosis indicated a normal distribution on all the variables. Discriminant function analysis was employed first on the high ($n = 220$) and low ($n = 218$) perceived stress groups for war and nonwar categories. Then a third discriminant function analysis was applied to the four groups noted in Table 6.1. Predictors were physical health, psychological health, depression, and interpersonal and marital relationships.

Perceived War Stress

Based on stepwise discriminant function analysis, interpersonal relationship was the first predictor to be included ($F = 72.08$, $df = 1, 436$, $p < 0.0001$), followed by physical health ($F = 54.73$, $df = 1, 436$, $p < 0.0001$), and depression ($F = 40.64$, *df* = 1, 436, $p < 0.0001$). Psychological health and marital relations were dropped as predictors by the statistical criterion for inclusion in the equation. The canonical discriminant function (Table 6.3) with the three predictors in the equation accounted for 28% of the variance with an Eigen value of 0.28, canonical correlation = 0.47, and Wilks's Lambda = 0.78 ($\chi^2 = 107.58$ (3), $p < 0.0001$). The standardized canonical discriminant function coefficients were 0.39 for physical, 0.38 for depression, and 0.65 for interpersonal relationships.

The overall correct classification was 68.5%, with classification accuracy strong for both groups. Prediction was best in the low-stress group (73.9%), and 63.2% in the high-stress group (Table 6.5).

Perceived Nonwar Stress

Based on stepwise discriminant function analysis, all predictors were significant. Depression was the first predictor to be included ($F = 21.40$, *df* = 1, 436, $p < 0.0001$), followed by interpersonal relations ($F = 16.21$, *df* = 1, 436, $p < 0.0001$), marital relations ($F = 12.44$, *df* = 1, 436, $p < 0.0001$), physical health ($F = 10.55$, *df* = 1, 436, $p < 0.0001$), and psychological health ($F = 8.73$, *df* = 1, 436, $p < 0.0001$). The canonical discriminant function (Table 6.4) had an Eigen value of 0.10, canonical correlation = 0.303, and Wilks's Lambda = 908 ($\chi^2 = 41.7[5]$, $p < 0.0001$), suggesting that a significant difference existed between high and low nonwar stress groups on the predictor variables accounting for 10% of the variance.

The overall correct classification for nonwar stress was 63.7% (the average of high and low stress). Classification accuracy was strong for both groups; prediction was best in the low-stress group (68.8%), and 58.5% in the high-stress group (Table 6.5).

Perceived War And Nonwar Stress Groups

As described at the beginning of this section, cross-tabulation of high and low perceived war and nonwar stress, yielded four groups (Table 6.1). The group sizes

TABLE 6.3. Canonical Discriminant Function to Predict Membership in High and Low Perceived War Stress Groups

Function	Eigen Value	Canonical Correlation	λ	χ^2	*df*
After 0	0.283	0.497	0.779	108.04*	5

Standardized Variable	Canonical Discriminant Function Coefficient
Physical	0.39
Psychological	0.01
Depression	0.35
Interpersonal	0.62
Marital	0.09

*$p < .0001$.

TABLE 6.4. Canonical Discriminant Function to Predict Membership in High And Low Nonwar Stress Groups

Function	Eigen Value	Canonical Correlation	λ	χ^2	*df*
	0.10	0.303	0.908	41.7*	5

Standardized Variable	Canonical Discriminant Function Coefficient
Physical	0.47
Psychological	-0.24
Depression	0.38
Interpersonal	0.46
Marital	0.36

$^*p < .0001$.

TABLE 6.5. Classification Results in the High and Low War and Nonwar Stress Groups

Group	Cases	Predicted Group Membership: Low	Predicted Group Membership: High
War Stress Group			
Low	218	161 (73.9%)	57 (26.1%)
High	220	81 (36.8%)	139 (63.2%)
Nonwar Stress Group			
Low	221	152 (68.8%)	69 (31.2%)
High	217	90 (41.5%)	127 (58.5%)

were 137 for high on both categories, 138 for low on both categories, 80 for high nonwar and low war, and 83 for high war and low nonwar perceived stress.

Based on stepwise discriminant function analysis on the four groups using five family adaptation variables as predictors of membership, interpersonal relationship was the first predictor to be included ($F = 27.01$, $df = 3, 434$, $p < .0001$), followed by physical health ($F = 20.56$, $df = 3, 434$, $p < 0.0001$), depression ($F = 15.06$, $df = 3, 434$, $p < 0.0001$), marital relations ($F = 12.09$, $df = 3, 434$, $p < 0.0001$). Psychological health did not enter the equation ($F = .51$, $df = 3, 434$, $p > 0.05$).

The canonical discriminant function (Table 6.6) had an Eigen value of 0.34, canonical correlation = 0.503, Wilks's Lambda = 0.729 ($\chi^2 = 138.5[15]$, $p < 0.0001$). The standardized canonical discriminant function coefficients were 0.58 for interpersonal relationships, 0.43 for physical, 0.37 for depression, 0.17 for marital, and 0.05 for psychological, respectively (see Table 6.6).

TABLE 6.6. Canonical Discriminant Function to Predict Membership in High and Low War and Nonwar Stress Groups

Function	Eigen Value	Canonical Correlation	λ	χ^2	*df*
	0.34	0.503	0.726	138.5*	15

Standardized Variable	Canonical Discriminant Function Coefficient
Physical	0.43
Depression	0.37
Interpersonal	0.58
Marital	0.17

$^*p < .0001$.

Table 6.7 displays classification results from the discriminant function analysis for high- and low-stress families in the perceived war and nonwar groups. The overall correct classification in the four groups was 41.55%. However, when psychological health was removed from the equation, overall prediction improved to 44% and to 51% in the high and 60% in the low groups. Classification accuracy was stronger in the extreme (groups 1 and 2) than in the combination groups (3 and 4). Prediction was best (55.1%) in the low-stress group, followed by 49.6% in the high-stress group, 17.5% and 28.9% in groups 3 and 4, respectively. Findings indicated a high degree of consistency in the prediction and classification scheme especially in the high- and low-stress groups in all of the above categories (Table 6.7 displays these results).

In view of these results, the study hypothesis was supported. The low-stress groups indicated more positive adaptation than the high-stress groups in all categories of the perceived war and nonwar life events and a combination of the two.

DISCUSSION

This study was concerned with comparing high- and low-stress Lebanese families on the basis of their perceived life events with respect to war and nonwar stressors and to identify a set of predictors that can discriminate between high- and low-stress families. The hypothesis predicted that, based on their perceived life events score (war, nonwar, and a combination of the two), the low-stress group would indicate more positive adaptation, as reflected by physical health, psychological health, depression, and interpersonal and marital relationships.

Study findings showed that interpersonal relationships, physical health, and depression were the best predictors of membership in the high/low war stress groups. In the perceived nonwar stress groups, depression, interpersonal relationships, marital relations, and physical and psychological health were the best

TABLE 6.7. Classification Results in the High and Low War and Nonwar Perceived Stress Groups

Actual Group	Cases	Predicted Group Membership 1	2	3	4
Group 1	137	68.0	22.0	17.0	30.0
		49.6%	16.1%	12.4%	21.9%
Group 2	138	13.0	76.0	32.0	17.0
		9.4%	55.1%	23.2%	12.3%
Group 3	80	14.0	32.0	14.0	20.0
		0.5%	40.0%	17.5%	25.0%
Group 4	83	23.0	15.0	21.0	24.0
		27.7%	18.1%	25.3%	28.9%

Groups: (1) = high war and nonwar stress; (2) = low war and nonwar stress; (3) = high nonwar, low war; (4) = high war, low nonwar.

predictors separating high/low stress groups. When the combination scores of war and nonwar stress was used, interpersonal relationships, physical health, depression, and marital relations were the best predictors distinguishing among the groups.

Findings indicated a high degree of consistency in the prediction and classification of the high/low stress groups and for all stress categories. Families in the low-stress groups had a more positive adaptation than those in the high-stress groups and could be classified on the basis of their stress score. Family adaptation was assessed in terms of physical and psychological health, depression, and interpersonal and marital relationships. Thus family adaptation was higher in families reporting lower symptoms in the areas of physical and mental health, depression, and interpersonal and marital relationships; families who perceived low war and nonwar stress fared better than those in the high-stress groups on their physical and mental health outcomes, and in their relationship with the spouse and others. The reverse also holds. For example, families with lower levels of symptoms and higher level of satisfaction with their relationships tended to perceive lower levels of war and nonwar stress than those in high-stress category. Families in the high-stress groups had more complaints than their counterparts in the low-stress groups. This is an important finding in explaining and predicting family adaptation. This classification could serve in identifying why some families are better able to adapt to stressful situations than others. Findings of this study support the association between perceived stress and family health and interactional outcomes. Perceived war and nonwar stress negatively affect perceived physical, mental, interpersonal, and marital well-being. This finding is in line with Olson and McCubbin's (1989) conceptualization on family well-being, also with Holmes and Masuda's (1974) work that links the accumulation of life events to onset of illness: The greater the magnitude of life events, the greater the risk of illness and the greater the seriousness of the illness.

Although there is a growing body of knowledge in the area of family stress and health outcomes, no account of classifying families into high- and low-stress groups has been reported in the literature. McCubbin and Patterson (1983) developed the Typology Model of Family Adjustment and Adaptation. Family types were classified over the life cycle; adaptability depended on certain aspects consistent with a particular stage. McCubbin and McCubbin (1987) introduced the T-Double ABCX Model of Family Adjustment and Adaptation. The model focused on normative and family transitions and life cycle stage. With such a different focus, comparison of results seems inadequate.

However, the present findings seem to support the growing body of literature and the great demand for classifying families into high- and low-stress groups. This is in line with Olson and McCubbin's (1989) findings that individuals and families with more problems would tend to fall at the extremes of the cohesion and adaptability dimensions. Conceptually, findings of this study enable us to incorporate change strategies that are needed for intervention within a framework that takes perception of life events and stressors into account. Such conceptualization incorporates family hardships and accumulation demands from all areas of family life inherent in chronic crisis such as those arising from prolonged war situations. Family classification into unique and distinct groups helps us characterize how families function and adapt. This may prove helpful to mental health professionals in their effort to understand how families negotiate change and adapt in response to stressful situations. Additionally, findings of this study build and add on the previous findings (Farhood, 1999) in that we know more than predicting paths and aspects of the model. The present findings tell us about family adaptation outcome in the face of stress and shed light into how families with high stress succumb to mental, relational, and emotional stress. Mental health professionals are urged to identify vulnerable families and understand how families adapt in response to normative and nonnormative life events.

REFERENCES

American Psychiatric Association. (2000). *Diagnostic and statistical manual of mental disorders* (4th ed.). Washington, DC: Author.

Beck, A. T., & Steer, R. A. (1993). *Beck Depression Inventory Manual.* San Antonio, TX: Harcourt Brace.

Bryce, J., Walker, N., Ghorayeb, F., & Kanj, M. (1989). Life experiences, responses styles and mental health among mothers and children in Beirut, Lebanon. *Social Science and Medicine, 28,* 685-695.

Burr, W. R. (1973). *Theory construction and the sociology of the family.* New York: John Wiley and Sons.

Farhood, L., & Noureddine, S. (2003). PTSD, depression and health status in Lebanese civilians exposed to a church explosion. *International Journal of Psychiatry in Medicine, 33*(1), 39-53.

Farhood, L. (1999). War and nonwar stressors, family resources, coping and family adaptation among Lebanese families. *Archives of Psychiatric Nursing, 13*(4), 192-203.

Farhood, L., Zurayk, H., Chaaya, M., Saadeh, F., Meshefedjian, G., & Sidani, T. (1993). The impact of war on physical and mental health of the family: The Lebanese experience. *Social Science and Medicine, 36*(12), 1555-1567.

Feetham, S. (1991). Conceptual and methodological issues in research of families. In A. L. Whall & J. Fawcett, *Family theory development in nursing: State of the science and art.* Philadelphia: F. A. Davis Co.

Garrison, C., Bryant, E., Addy, C., Spurrier, P., Freedy, J., & Kilpatrick, D. (1995). Posttraumatic stress in adolescents after Hurricane Andrew. *Journal of American Academy of Child and Adolescent Psychiatry, 34*(9), 1193-1201.

Garrity, T. F., & Marx, M. B. (1985). Effects of moderator variables on the response to stress. In S. R. Burchfield (Ed.), *Stress: Psychological and physiological interactions.* Washington, DC: Hemisphere Publishing.

Goenjian, A. K., Naganian, M., Pynoos, R. S., Steinberg, A. M., Mamoukian, G., Tavosian, A., & Fairbanks, L. A. (1994). Post-traumatic stress disorder in elderly and younger adults after the 1988 earthquake in Armenia. *American Journal of Psychiatry, 151,* 895-901.

Green, B. L. (1994). Psychological research in traumatic stress: An update. *Journal of Traumatic Stress, 17,* 341-362.

Hardin, S. B., Weinrich, M., Weinrich, S., Hardin, T. L., & Garrison, C. (1994). Psychological distress of adolescents exposed to Hurricane Hugo. *Journal of Traumatic Stress, 7,* 427-440.

Hill, R. (1949). *Families under stress.* New York: Harper.

Hill, R. (1958). Generic features of families under stress. *Social Casework, 49,* 139-150.

Holmes, T. H., & Masuda, M. (1974). Life change and illness susceptibility. In B. S. Dohrenwend & B. P. Dohrenwend (Eds.), *Stressful life events.* New York: Wiley.

Holmes, T. H., & Rahe, R. H. (1967). The social readjustment rating scale. *Journal of Psychosomatic Research, II,* 213-218.

Kaplan, G. A., Roberts, R. E., Camacho, T. C., & Coyne, J. C. (1987). Psychosocial predictors of depression: Prospective evidence from the human population laboratory studies. *American Journal of Epidemiology, 125*(2), 206-220.

Karam, E., & Bou Ghosn, M. (2003). Psychological consequences of war among civilian populations. *Current Opinion in Psychiatry, 16,* 413-419.

Lipman-Blumen, J. (1975). A crisis framework applied to macrosociological family change, marriage, divorce, and occupational trends associated with World War II. *Journal of Marriage and the Family, 27,* 889-902.

McCubbin, H., Joy, D., Cauble, J., Patterson, J., & Needle, R. (1980). Family stress, coping and social support: A decade review. *Journal of Marriage and the Family, 42,* 855-871.

McCubbin, M., & McCubbin, H. (1987). *Family assessment inventories for research practice.* Madison: University of Wisconsin.

McCubbin, H. I., & Patterson J. M. (1983). The family stress process: The Double ABCX model of family adjustments and adaptation. In H. I. McCubbin, M. Sussman, & J. Patterson (Eds.), *Advances and developments in family stress theory and Research.* New York: Haworth.

Olson, D., & McCubbin, H. I. (1989). *Families.* Newbury Park, CA: Sage.

Pearlin, L. I., Liberman, M. A., Menaghan, E. G., & Mullan, J. T. (1981). The stress process. *Journal of Health and Social Behavior, 22,* 337-356.

Persson, M., Runeson, B., & Wasserman, D. (1999). Diagnosis, psychosocial stressors and adaptive functioning in attempted suicide. *Annals of Clinical Psychiatry, 11*(3), 119-128.

Rotter, J. B. (1966). Generalized expectancies for internal versus external control of reinforcement. *Psychological Monographs, 80*(1), 1-28.

Saab, B. R., Chaaya, M., Doumit, M., & Farhood, L. (2003). Predictors of psychological distress in Lebanese hostages of war. *Social Science and Medicine, 57,* 1249-1257.

Schlenger, W. E., Caddely, M., & Elbert, L. (2002). Psychological reactions to terrorist attacks. *Journal of the American Medical Association, 288,* 581-588.

Sha'ar, K., & Bryce, J. (1986). Description of the research. In J. Bryce & H. Armenian (Eds.), *In wartime: The state of children in Lebanon.* Beirut, Lebanon: American University of Beirut Press.

Zegans, L. S. (1982). Stress and the development of somatic disorders. In L. Goldburger & S. Breznitz (Eds.), *Handbook of stress: Theoretical and clinical aspects.* New York: The Free Press.

Zurayk, H., & Armenian, H. (Eds.). (1985). *Beirut 1984: A population and health profile.* Beirut, Lebanon: American University of Beirut.

Acknowledgments. This study was funded by the University Research Board at the American University of Beirut, grant number 116010-48101. The author would like to thank Dr. Elizabeth Lenz, Ohio State University, and Dr. Karen Soeken, University of Maryland, Baltimore, for their support throughout this work. Special thanks go to the families who participated in the study.

7

Chronic Stress Conditions Do Explain Posttraumatic Brain Injury Depression

Esther Bay
Ned Kirsch
Brenda Gillespie

Traumatic brain injury (TBI) is a significant public health concern throughout the world and often referred to as the silent epidemic because the resulting problems are not always visible (Centers for Disease Control, 1999). Nearly 1.5 million new cases of brain injury occur each year (Mooney & Speed, 2001), and about 5.3 million Americans are disabled from brain injury. Over three-fourths of those with hospital admission for brain injury consist of those sustaining mild-to-moderate brain injury (Levin, Williams, Eisenberg, High, & Guinto, 1992). Moderate head injury affects approximately 75,000 Americans each year, two thirds experiencing moderate disability (Goldstein, 2003). According to the National Institutes of Health (NIH) Consensus Report, annual costs associated with this population are estimated to be in excess of $9 billion (Panel of the National Institutes of Health, 1999).

Depression, a common mood disorder after TBI, has a reported incidence up to 77% (Seel et al., 2003). The presence of depression leads to indifference and lack of motivation to participate in much needed, yet limited rehabilitation therapies. Depression is exhibited regardless of the severity of injury, has a protracted course, adds to cognitive difficulty, and most likely contributes to substance abuse and family discord (Atteberry-Bennett, Barth, Loyd, & Lawrence, 1986; Levin et al., 2001; Ownsworth & Oei, 1998; Seel et al., 2003). Head injury during early adulthood increases the lifetime prevalence for major depressive disorder (Holsinger et al., 2002).

Explanations for post-TBI depression are largely atheoretical and remain unclear (Ownsworth & Oei, 1998). Some empirical findings indicate depression is explained by an organic malady, physical health impairment, or psychosocial variables such as reduced financial status (Fann, Katon, Uomoto, & Esselman, 1995; Jorge, Robinson, Arndt, Forrester, et al., 1993; Kinsella, Moran, Ford, & Ponsford, 1988; McCleary et al., 1998; Seel et al., 2003). After mild-to-moderate TBI, depression is linked to posttraumatic stress disorder (PTSD; Levin et al., 2001).

The study of post-TBI depression is limited by the lack of theoretically focused variables that are amenable to interventions. McEwen's stress theory of allostasis is the guiding framework for this study and could become a framework for intervention studies (McEwen, 2002). The purpose of this study is to identify pre- and postinjury chronic stress conditions that are likely to contribute to post-TBI depressive symptoms.

BACKGROUND

Depressive symptoms create considerable distress and often produce similar functional limitations as major chronic health problems (Breslau & Davis, 1986; Wells et al., 1989). Depressive symptoms are associated with measures of self-esteem, hopelessness, and sadness and may represent the construct of demoralization, believed to accompany severe physical and psychological illness (Breslau & Davis, 1986).

Post-TBI depression research remains at the descriptive level with most focusing on the best measures and methods of measurement (Bay, 2000; Jorge, Robinson, Arndt, Forrester, et al., 1993; Kreutzer, Marwitz, Seel, & Serio, 1996; Kreutzer, Seel, & Gourley, 2001; Seel et al., 2003; Sliwinski, Gordon, & Bogdany, 1998). Kreutzer and associates developed a self-report instrument standardized with over 500 persons recovering from TBI that measured neurobehavioral functioning and depressed mood (Kreutzer et al., 1996). One subscale of the instrument consisted of 13 items measuring depressive symptoms and will be the dependent variable in this study because of its validity with persons who experienced TBI.

The ability to obtain reliable data about depressive symptoms from persons with TBI has also been highly debated because of variability in postinjury self-awareness. For those with mild-to-moderate TBI, the sample selected for this study, there is agreement that measures of self-report can be reliably obtained. These studies utilized relatives/significant others (R/SO) or therapists to also rate the persons' mood and behavioral state and noted no rating differences on mood or behavioral function (Bay, 2001; Kreutzer et al., 1996; McCleary et al., 1998). Therefore, it is expected that self-report data can be reliably obtained from the survivor.

The atheoretical status of post-TBI depression research and lack of focus on potential interventions is illustrated by the following studies. Jorge and associates asserted that post-TBI depression was associated with specific brain lesions located in the left anterior region of the frontal lobe (Jorge, Robinson, Arndt, Starkstein, et al., 1993). These same investigators also reported on depression onset in their 1-year longitudinal study and noted an acute and delayed onset (Jorge, Robinson, Arndt, Forrester, et al., 1993a). Another model examined the relationship between depression and overall functional outcome as measured with the Glasgow Outcome Scale score at 6 months (Satz et al., 1998) and 1 year postinjury (McCleary et al., 1998). Interestingly, there was a significant relationship between functional status and depression at six months, but this relationship was not present at the 1-year evaluation. Functional status, as measured with the Medical Health Outcomes Study Health Survey, was reported to be more impaired in those with depression in a total sample of 50 persons recruited from TBI outpatient clinics who were within 3 years of injury (Fann, Uomoto, & Katon, 2001). Seel and colleagues asserted that those reporting depression were more likely to have preinjury unemployment and postinjury financial loss (Seel et al., 2003).

Depression is related to chronic stress (Bay, Hagerty, Williams, Kirsch, & Gillespie, 2002; Breslau & Davis, 1986; Davidson et al., 2002; McEwen, 2002). Chronic stress is a pernicious biobehavioral state resulting from persistent demands of the environment or from an event or experience perceived as threatening or demanding because it produced an allostatic load on the person's physical or psychological capacity and precipitated a sequential chain of physical, emotional, cognitive, and interpersonal difficulties. Chronic stress most likely results when the survivor is confronted with financial difficulties, losses in relationships and personal identity, family discord, legal conflicts, daily hassles, treatment-related confinements, physical distress, and changes in independence. Responses to the chronic stress state include habituation, modification through the buffering effects of social support networks and helping professionals, increased perception of physical symptoms, substance abuse, and behavioral or interpersonal change, while others experience mood disorders such as depression (Breslau & Davis, 1986; Davidson et al., 2002; McEwen, 2002).

These difficulties are not uncommon to those with other chronic or uncertain medical conditions, but are experienced uniquely after TBI. Typically, the injured person is under age 35 and developmentally positioned for work and family responsibilities (Ownsworth & Oei, 1998). The event is unexpected, often associated with an accident, and the person's cognitive abilities are compromised. The time course of this chronic stress experience is unknown and there may be a preexisting chronic stress state prior to the injury that exacerbates the postinjury stress experience (Bay, 2000).

Preinjury and Postinjury Chronic Stress and Depressive Symptoms

Relationships between chronic stress and depression are well-established in the psychiatric literature (Anisman & Zacharko, 1992; Gold, Goodwin, & Chrousos, 1988; Nemeroff, 1998) and imply that stress and depression are more likely linked when there is a specific vulnerability factor (Post, 1992), such as the preexistence of childhood adversity (Kessler & Magee, 1993; Liu et al., 1997; Young, Abelson, Curtis, & Nesse, 1997) or major stressful life events (Cohen, Kessler, & Gordon, 1995; Schaeffer & Baum, 1984), or when the stress event is the basis for persistent threat appraisal resulting in significant lifestyle change and adjustment (Breslau & Davis, 1986).

Chronic stress before brain injury was investigated. Raskin (1997) examined the impact of preinjury chronic stress exposure (sexual abuse) on cognition and mood after minor brain injury (MBI) and concluded that chronic stress exposure resulted in significant deficits in executive function and working memory (Raskin, 1997). In an investigation of 100 consecutively admitted survivors, Bowen and associates found that those unemployed prior to injury and tested 6 months after the injury were more likely to have mood disorders (Bowen, Neumann, Conner, Tennant, & Chamberlain, 1998). Further, MBI survivors were more likely to display persistent postinjury difficulties when there were significant preinjury stressors (Fenton, McClelland, Montgomery, MacFlynn, & Rutherford, 1993; Rimel, Giordani, Barth, Boll, & Jane, 1981). Finally, an investigation of whether a major life event prior to stroke contributed to poststroke depression yielded results showing that there was a significant relationship between this prestroke chronic stress event and post-stroke depression, measured with the Center for Epidemiologic Studies-Depression Scale (CES-D; Bush, 1999).

Brain-injury theorists posited that chronic stress before and after injury impacts adjustment (Kendall & Terry, 1996; Malia, Powell, & Torode, 1995; Martelli, Zasler, & MacMillan, 1998). However, empirical testing of these propositions is not well published. Bay and associates reported that the frequency of perceived chronic stress after injury explained 58% of the variance in depressive symptoms and that lowered sense of belonging or a feeling of not being valued and fitting in explained nearly 60% of the variance in depressive symptoms (Bay et al., 2002). Levin and associates reported an association between posttraumatic stress disorder and major depression disorder in their sample of mild to moderate brain injured persons who were tested 3 months after the injury (Levin et al., 2001). Thus exposure to pre- and postinjury stressors may explain post-TBI depression.

Theory of Allostasis and Stress

McEwen's theory of stress and allostasis (McEwen, 2002) provides a new perspective for examining the impact stress has on the damaged and recovering brain. Stress is an external event with the potential for serious long-term consequences. An internal allostasis system equips one to deal with stress to preserve body integrity. Its function is to activate or deactivate the brain and supporting structures in order to withstand the body's demands. The allostatic system, primarily regulated by the brain, responds to physical states (e.g., exercise, hunger, arousal, and position changes), environment conditions (e.g., noise, crowding), and danger (e.g., trauma or abuse). This response is mediated by the person's state of physical health and perception of the stress event.

Given a stress event, the primary response is to activate the sympathetic nervous system and hypothalamic-pituitary-adrenal (HPA) axis. This HPA axis can effectively orchestrate balance between the nervous system, glands, and immune system by activating cortisol secretion or inhibiting its release with receptors located in the hippocampus. Still, prolonged underactivity or overactivity of the allostatic system, termed allostatic load, can impair its function. Allostatic load, if prolonged, contributes to disease states such as depression, memory impairment, substance abuse, and other stress-related diseases.

Preinjury or postinjury stress conditions may sensitize the person to or produce allostatic load after injury. Preinjury stress conditions found to contribute to postinjury difficulties with cognition or depression include exposure to sexual abuse (Raskin, 1997) or preinjury social adversities (Fenton et al., 1993; Rimel et al., 1981). Postinjury stress conditions contributing to allostatic load include those associated with stressful life events, daily hassles, or chronic stress associated with the brain injury event. Perceived chronic stress is most likely an indicator of allostatic load.

Thus, this study examined relationships between pre- and postinjury chronic stress, and post-TBI depression using McEwen's framework of allostasis as the guidepost. Using a cross-sectional survey design, the following hypotheses were tested:

Hypothesis 1. There is a significant and positive relationship between preinjury stressors and post-TBI depressive symptoms.

Hypothesis 2. There is a significant and positive relationship between pre- and postinjury chronic stress and TBI depressive symptoms.

METHODS

The sample consisted of 75 survivors with mild-to-moderate levels of brain injury who were admitted to the hospital at the time of injury, were within 2 years of their injury at the time of testing, and were evaluated and treated by brain injury specialists in five outpatient rehabilitation centers affiliated with large urban teaching centers with specialties in trauma care. Persons were excluded if they were psychotic at the time of testing, had a preinjury neurological impairment, could not speak or understand English, and were not between 18 and 65 years of age. Institutional Review Board approval was obtained from the authors' affiliated institution, as well as from the five brain-injury clinics. While exact numbers are unknown, approximately 125 additional persons from these five clinics met the eligibility criteria for the study, but refused to participate because they were "too busy," "too stressed," or "tired of answering questions and not getting any answers."

Former rehabilitation center participants who met the eligibility criteria were invited by letter to participate and received a follow-up phone call to ascertain that they received the letter, while all newly admitted survivors meeting the eligibility criteria were given a letter of invitation to participate. Data collection occurred over 15 months (July 1999 to September 2000), and ceased when 75 TBI participants were enrolled.

After informed and signed consent, the survivor selected a relative/significant other (R/SO) participant to provide supplemental data and chose a location, date, and time for the data collection. While it was estimated that the data collection period would occur over a single 60-minute testing period, accommodations were made for survivor fatigue, therapy scheduling conflicts, and transportation difficulties. The sequence of testing was consistent for all participants. Data were collected in the presence of the principal investigator. No participant's data were excluded from the analyses; therefore, no data were discarded due to incomplete responses. To increase the reliability that retrospective data about the duration of unconsciousness (LOC) and length of posttraumatic amnesia (PTA) were accurate, both the R/SO and survivor were asked questions regarding brain injury severity.

DEMOGRAPHIC AND MEASUREMENT RESULTS

On the date of testing, 30 survivors were within 7 months of their injury, and 45 were between 7 and 25 months from the date of injury. On average, the survivor was assessed 9.57 months after the date of injury (*SD* = 6.31). Nearly 71% of the sample received the TBI as a result of a motor vehicle crash, while 13.3% experienced a fall and 12% experienced a pedestrian/auto accident. The remaining sample incurred the brain injury because of violence or a sports injury. The sample was predominately Caucasian, for the only minority represented was African American and included 9.3% of the sample. Forty-eight percent of the sample were women. The average age was 37.4 years (*SD* = 12.10, range 19-60). Thirty-six percent were never married, 40% were married, and 20% were divorced, separated, or widowed. Four percent were living with a significant other. One third reported annual household incomes in excess of $75,000, and 14.7% reported annual incomes below $15,000.

Overall, 65% rated themselves to be in good to excellent health at the time of testing. Thirteen percent had been previously treated for alcohol or drug problems. Forty-one percent were taking prescribed antidepressants, but no data were collected on the drug, dosage, and duration, nor were data collected about DSM-IV diagnosis at the time of testing. Nearly 7% reported not having filled prescriptions for antidepressants. Twenty percent reported preinjury psychiatric disorders, such as anxiety or depression, 8% said they had suicidal thoughts the year prior to the injury, and 16% had a previous head injury. No one was involved in the accident because of a suicide attempt. Despite nearly 41% of the sample taking antidepressant medications, participants reported higher levels of depressive symptoms.

Estimates of Brain Injury Severity. Traditional measures were used to determine brain injury severity: Glasgow Coma Scale (GCS) score, PTA, and duration of LOC. The GCS score used was the admitting score received by the participant as evaluated by nurses and physicians during the emergency admission. If a person was labeled as a score of 3 because of sedation or substance use intoxication and the next awakening score was > 8, that person was eligible for the study. The duration of PTA and LOC was difficult to obtain and the information was only included when chart data were clear about this or when the investigator could obtain reliable data from the R/SO.

During questioning about the duration of PTA, the R/SO was asked to recall when the person began making reliable, continuous basic memories. Using chart review, these measures were used to classify those with mild brain injury (MBI) according to the definition established by the 1993 American Congress of Rehabilitation Medicine (ACRM): PTA < 24 hours and LOC < 30 minutes and GCS of 13 to 15 (ACRM,

1993). An exception to the ACRM definition was made for those who had a GCS of 13 to 15 and an abnormal computed tomography (CT) report. They were classified as moderately injured (Satz et al., 1998). Persons classified with moderate brain injury also had a duration of LOC exceeding 30 minutes but less than 2 weeks, PTA > 24 hours, and an admission GCS score of 9 to 12.

Those with a mild or moderate injury were equally represented. The average duration of PTA, determined with chart review or questioning the survivor or relative/significant other, was 7.65 days (SD = 8.92, range 0-45 days). Slightly more than 48% had abnormal CT results, showing small hemorrhages, hematomas, or contusions. The anatomical location of the injury was not recorded. Nearly 71% reported that a motor vehicle crash was the mechanism of injury and 64% reported the duration of unconsciousness to be brief to less than an hour.

Depressive Symptoms. The depression subscale of the Neurobehavioral Functioning Inventory (NFI), a 76-item self-report inventory defining problems currently experienced by persons with neurological injury (Kreutzer, Seel, & Marwitz, 1999), was used as the dependent variable. It consists of 13 items with ratings on a 5-point Likert scale that sum to scores between 13 and 65 and shows construct validity with the Minnesota Multiphasic Personality Inventory (MMPI) depression scale (r = .47). Criterion-related validity and high internal consistency are reported in the NFI manual (Kreutzer et al., 1999). In this study, the Cronbach's alpha coefficient for depressive symptoms was .92, range 13 to 54, and the mean was 30.69 (SD = 10.66). Results indicated a significant and positive correlation between depression and time-since-injury (r = .388, p = .001).

Chronic Stress. To determine the presence of preinjury stress, the survivor was asked to complete two checklists asking whether the event did or did not occur. The Childhood Adversity Checklist (CAC) was a 16-item checklist modified from a questionnaire developed by Kupfer and colleagues (Cohen, Coyne, & Duvall, 1993; Kupfer & Detre, 1974). It asked whether specific circumstances affecting their family relationships occurred during childhood, such as family violence, drinking, or abuse. Secondly, a 12-item checklist adapted from the Holmes and Rahe Scale of Stressful Life Events (SLE) quantified the frequency of specific stressful events occurring within 6 months prior to the brain injury. Participants endorsed each event with a yes or no response. These items correlate highly with the onset of depression (Cohen et al., 1995). For this study, the R/SO was invited to review this particular list with the survivor to enhance accuracy in the responses. Responses on the CAC ranged from 0 to 10, mean = 3.67 (SD = 2.78). Responses on the SLE Checklist ranged from 0 to 6, M = 1.52 (SD = 1.54).

Postinjury stress was measured with the Perceived Stress Scale (PSS), a 14-item Likert measure of global stress encountered over the past 30 days (Cohen, Kamarck, & Mermelstein, 1983). This measure correlates with the CES-D and Beck Depression Inventory (BDI; r = .70) and has good reliability (α = .85; Cohen et al., 1995). Williams and associates reported the average PSS for those with depression (measured with the BDI) and living in the community was 33.7 (Williams et al., 2000). For this investigation, the range was 5 to 52 (M = 28.36, SD = 9.45) and alpha coefficient was .87.

RESULTS

Hypothesis 1. This hypothesis examined the relationship between preinjury stressors and post-TBI depression. The responses on the CAC portrayed persons whose childhoods were filled with turmoil. Nearly 50% reported a prevalence of financial difficulties during their childhood. Thirty-two percent reported drug or alcohol problems within the home and nearly 38% reported divorces during childhood. Three were sexually abused while 27% reported physical or verbal abuse from parents. Slightly more than 18% reported violence between their parents. Nearly 50% experienced the death of a family member during their childhood and 21% reported that their parents or caregivers had a significant chronic illness, such as mental illness, cancer, or alcoholism.

Results on the SLE checklist were quite varied. Nearly 22% had a friend or family member die within 6 months prior to the injury. Ten percent reported a marital separation prior to the injury and nearly 27% reported having significant difficulties with relatives 6 months prior. Sixteen percent admitted to having financial difficulties prior to the accident. Anecdotally, about 10% verbalized they encountered stressful life events after their injury, but no quantitative data were collected on this postinjury occurrence.

A series of regression models was constructed with the NFI-D depressive symptom score as the outcome variable. Initially, two preinjury stress variables were summed as indicators of preinjury allostatic load and simultaneously regressed on depressive symptoms. There were no significant findings. Then, each preinjury stress variable was entered into a regression model with depressive symptoms and again there were no significant relationships. Gender was not a significant variable in explaining depression in these models. Thus, these preinjury stress conditions did not collectively or individually explain variation in depressive symptoms after TBI.

Because time-since-injury was related to depressive symptoms in this study (Adjusted $R^2 = .14$, $F = 12.97$ [1, 73] , $p = .001$), this variable was entered with the summed preinjury stress conditions and important relationships were evident (see Table 7.1). A positive and significant relationship existed between the frequency of preinjury events, time-since-injury and depressive symptoms. Thus, hypothesis 1 was supported when time-since-injury was in the model. For every one standard

TABLE 7.1. Regression of NFI-D on Preinjury Stress and Time-Since-Injury*

Model	Unstandardized Coefficients		Standardized Coefficients		
	B	*SE*	*b*	*t*	*p*
Preinjury Stress	1.002	.328	.321	3.06	.003
Time-Since-Injury	.78	.18	.46	4.40	.000

*ANOVA results: Adjusted $R^2 = .23$, $F = 11.91$ (2, 72), $p = .000$.

deviation in preinjury stress, there was a .32 standard deviation increase in postinjury depression.

Hypothesis 2. This hypothesis examined whether pre- and postinjury chronic stress were related to post-TBI depression. Postinjury stress alone explained 54% of the variance in depressive symptoms (Adjusted $R^2 = .54$, $F = 87.72$ [1, 73], $p = .000$). Relationships between pre- and postinjury chronic stress, time-since-injury and depressive symptoms were examined with multiple regression models. The sum of preinjury childhood adversity and major stressful life events were simultaneously entered with postinjury chronic stress and the preinjury variables were not significant, yet when time-since-injury was in the model all variables were significant (Adjusted $R^2 = .67$, $F = 49.98$, [3, 71], $p = .000$). Both preinjury childhood adversity and major stressful life events were significant in explaining variability in depression when entered separately with postinjury stress and time-since-injury, but when entered collectively, childhood adversity was the only preinjury stress variable that achieved significance in explaining depressive symptoms (see Table 7.2).

Because the frequency of childhood adversity was a significant preinjury stress condition, when entered with postinjury stress and time-since-injury (Adjusted $R^2 = .65$, $F = 47.36$, [3, 71], $p = .000$), further analysis was required. To better discern the main and interaction effects, the Childhood Adversity and PSS variables were centered, an interaction term constructed, and depressive symptoms were regressed on these variables. While approaching significance, there was not a significant interaction of childhood adversity and postinjury stress (see Table 7.3). In addition, when the interaction term constructed with stressful life events and postinjury stress were examined with time-since-injury and postinjury stress, no interaction could be discerned.

DISCUSSION

As a result of this study, explanations for post-TBI depression are extended. This study does support propositions of TBI theorists and demonstrates linkages between post-TBI depression and chronic stress. Specifically, the existence of preinjury

TABLE 7.2. Regression of NFI-D on Pre- and Postinjury Stress and Time-Since-Injury*

	Unstandardized Coefficients		Standardized Coefficients		
Model	*B*	*SE*	*b*	*t*	*p*
Childhood Adversity	.578	0.26	.151	2.18	.041
Stressful Life Events	.869	0.52	.125	1.68	.103
Perceived Stress Scale	.751	0.78	.666	9.56	.000
Time-Since-Injury	.624	0.12	.369	5.02	.000

*ANOVA results: Adjusted $R^2 = .66$, $F = 37.13$ (4, 70), $p = .000$.

TABLE 7.3. Regression of NFI-D on Interaction of Childhood Adversity, Postinjury Stress and Time-Since-Injury*

Model	Unstandardized Coefficients		Standardized Coefficients		
	B	*SE*	*b*	*t*	*p*
Preinjury Stress	1.002	.328	.321	3.06	.003
Childhood Adversity**	0.79	.28	.21	2.80	.000
Post Injury Stress**	0.77	.09	.67	9.05	.000
Time-Since-Injury	0.52	.12	.31	4.22	.000
Childhood × Postinjury Stress**	.01	.03	.13	1.80	.081

*ANOVA results: Adjusted $R^2 = .60$, $F = 30.37$ (4, 70), $p = .000$.
**Reflects centered variables.

childhood adversity and postinjury perceived stress were important explanatory variables in this cross-sectional study. Finally, there was support that given both a preinjury stress condition with postinjury stress, there is most likely allostatic load, for 65% of the variance in depression was explained by childhood adversity, time-since-injury, and postinjury stress.

From this study, it is evident that preinjury stress with time-since-injury added to the regression models does explain some variation in depressive symptoms after TBI. This finding supports a potential vulnerability factor for post-TBI depression and lends support for a sensitization mechanism. Conceptualizing childhood adversities and major stressful life events as a vulnerability condition for adult-onset depression is empirically rooted within the psychiatric literature (Anisman & Zacharko, 1982; Ladd, Owens, & Nemeroff, 1996; Nemeroff, 1998). Theorists and researchers concerned with post-TBI mood disorders also report that preinjury stress load is important in adjustment to the injury (Kendall & Terry, 1996; Ownsworth & Oei, 1998; Raskin, 1997). Further, this preinjury stress condition may disrupt the balance of allostasis, promote allostatic load, and contribute to negative outcomes, such as depression.

Further, Post (1992) proposed a theory of sensitization in explaining the relationship between stress and major depression. This theorist provided evidence that overwhelming psychosocial stressors were capable of instituting an acute onset depression and offered supporting evidence that subsequent, repetitive, albeit milder stressors, had the capacity to initiate neuroplastic change. Thus, continued or repetitive stress exposures alter brain structures and may contribute to neuroplastic change or brain damage leading to negative outcomes.

Sensitization was presented as a potential explanation for MBI depression, yet further testing of this conjecture is required (Busch & Alpern, 1998). Further, given the presence of significant childhood adversities with this population, and the subsequent likelihood that attachments and social connections are dysfunctional, there is increased likelihood that adult relationships may falter when a stressful event such as brain injury is encountered. Results from this study provide a basis for further longitudinal efforts regarding the patterns of change in social relationships as they impact post-TBI depression.

While this study was only cross-sectional, it is reasonable to conclude that postinjury stress and depressive symptoms are strongly and clearly related. Results from the present study support findings from those of Breslau and Davis (1986). The brain injury event resulted in multiple postinjury stresses: unemployment and thereby reduced income, multiple physical problems requiring numerous medical evaluations, cognitive decline, changes in social relationships (Bay, Hagerty, Williams, Kirsh, & Gillespie, 2002), and for some marital separation and divorce.

Thus, chronic stress conditions do impact depression and may be amenable to nursing interventions. Efforts to reduce the allostatic load on the brain, proposed to contribute to further brain damage (McEwen, 2002; Sapolsky, 1996), may be employed in early screening interviews by case managers or clinical specialists in neurology clinics. Further, nurses involved in case management or family support networks may be assistive in mediating the effects of chronic stress through education, stress management practices, or identifying those in need of close follow-up for overwhelming stress. Clearly, this study as depicted within the theory of allostasis could become a guide for intervention studies and for the practicing nurse.

Still, the limitations and strengths of this study need to be delineated. The sample was somewhat older, predominately Caucasian, and consisted of equal representation of men and women. The NIH Consensus report stated the average age of TBI survivors to be 15 to 24 or greater than age 75, and a predominately male population (Panel of the National Institutes of Health, 1999). Jorge and associates' study (Jorge, Robinson, Arndt, Forrester, et al., 1993) included largely third decade male volunteers with a history of substance abuse, while Satz and colleagues' (1998) study collected data with an 83% male sample (Satz et al., 1998).

Gender differences between the major study variables were not present, except on the PSS variable. Using *t*-test analysis for independent samples, females reported significantly higher postinjury stress ($t = 2.21$, $p = .03$). The fact there were no gender differences on levels of depression was surprising given the higher incidence of community depression among the female gender (Nolen-Hoeksema, 1987) and reports of greater degrees of Post-Concussion Syndrome in women, a diagnosis that may include those with depression (McCauley, Boake, Levin, Contant, & Song, 2001). It is unclear why women reported greater frequencies of postinjury stress when compared to men, as this was the only major study variable with a notable gender difference.

This sample closely resembled characteristics of other studies concerned with psychosocial variables. For example, 20% of the sample had a preinjury history of psychiatric disorder, typically reported as depression or anxiety, comparable to that reported by Jorge and associates (Jorge, Robinson, Arndt, Starkstein, et al., 1993). Sixteen percent admitted to a previous brain injury commonly sustained as a child, and one subject admitted to more than one brain injury, a finding reported by other researchers (Dikmen & Levin, 1993).

The measures and methods used to collect data were internally consistent, reliable, and valid. The study variables demonstrated Cronbach alphas in excess of

.85. Data were collected in the presence of the investigator. A recent study using the NFI as the measure of depression reported that this subscale closely approximates DSM-IV criteria (Seel et al., 2003). For this study, 33.4% reported feeling hopeless, 28% reported feeling worthless, while 58.7 % reported feeling sad. Nearly 42% described feelings of anhedonia, and 64% reported thoughts of rumination.

In this study, time-since-injury was an important variable in explaining depressed symptoms after brain injury. This finding was supported in other studies when investigators reported a decline in emotional functioning after the first 6 months of recovery, a time that often represents a depletion of resources and declines in attention and care from well-meaning friends and relatives (Jorge, Robinson, Arndt, Starkstein, et al., 1993; McCleary et al., 1998). They speculated that psychosocial factors accounted for this result.

As community reintegration occurs, there is awareness of multiple loss and notable decline in social contacts with medical personnel, friends, and coworkers while the array of permanent obstacles is often realized. These realizations may partly explain the relationship between depression and time-since-injury. In the present study, 91% reported being employed prior to the injury, while less than 50% were employed at the time of the assessment. Further, 2 participants were divorced during the hospitalization period, while 1 was widowed. When time-since-injury was recoded into "early" after injury, or within the first 6 months, as described by Jorge and associates, and "late," or those between 7 and 24 months postinjury (Jorge, Robinson, Arndt, Forrester, et al., 1993), the postinjury stress levels did not differ significantly, while the latter group were significantly more depressed ($t = 2.32$ [1, 73], $p = .02$).

These results can only be generalized to survivors with mild-to-moderate brain injury who were hospitalized and treated in outpatient brain-injury centers. The sample was a nonprobability sample and anyone meeting the eligibility criteria could participate. One could speculate that there was self-selection bias, yet the consent requested participation from those with and without depression. Further, the sample size is comparable to other published studies on depression and is adequately powered to show a medium effect for regression analysis with four independent variables (Cohen, 1992).

CONCLUSIONS

Psychosocial factors do contribute to post-TBI depression. The presence of preinjury childhood adversity may be a vulnerability factor contributing to allostatic load resulting in increased likelihood of depression after such a stress-producing event. How the adversity contributes to post-TBI depression requires further study. Perceived postinjury stress is clearly related to post-TBI depression and requires further deliberation over time, because as a measure of global chronic stress, it most likely measures perceived stress related to the event and daily hassles, as well as the physical changes and losses. A repeated measures design using this global stress measure would be appropriate. Additionally, there is a need to study the impact of stressful life events occurring after the injury and their relationship to post-TBI depression. Study of these variables over time with persons recovering from brain injury and comparing these results to a non-brain-injury control group is indicated.

REFERENCES

American Congress of Rehabilitation Medicine. (1993). Definition of mild traumatic brain injury. *Journal of Head Trauma Rehabilitation, 8*(3), 86-87.

Anisman, H., & Zacharko, R. (1982). Depression: The predisposing influence of stress. *The Behavioral and Brain Sciences, 5,* 89-106.

Anisman, H., & Zacharko, R. (1992). Depression as a consequence of inadequate neurochemical adaptation in response to stressors. *British Journal of Psychiatry, 160* (Suppl. 15), 36-43.

Atteberry-Bennett, J., Barth, J. T., Loyd, B., & Lawrence, E. (1986). The relationship between behavioral and cognitive deficits, demographics and depression in patients with minor head injuries. *International Journal of Clinical Neuropsychology, 8,* 114-117.

Bay, E. (2000). The biobehavioral correlates of post-traumatic brain injury depression. *Journal of Neuroscience Nursing, 32*(3), 169-176.

Bay, E. (2001). *Chronic stress, cortisol regulation, interpersonal relatedness, cognitive burden and depressive symptoms among community-dwelling survivors of brain injury.* Unpublished doctoral dissertation, University of Michigan, Ann Arbor.

Bay, E., Hagerty, B., Williams, R., Kirsch, N. & Gillespie, B. (2002). Chronic stress, sense of belonging, and depression among survivors of traumatic brain injury. *Journal of Nursing Scholarship* (Third quarter), 221-225.

Bowen, A., Neumann, V., Conner, M., Tennant, A., & Chamberlain, M. A. (1998). Mood disorders following traumatic brain injury: Identifying the extent of the problem and the people at risk. *Brain Injury, 12*(3), 177-190.

Breslau, N., & Davis, G. (1986). Chronic stress and major depression. *Archives of General Psychiatry, 43*(4), 309-314.

Busch, C., & Alpern, H. (1998). Depression after mild traumatic brain injury: A review of current research. *Neuropsychology Review, 8*(2), 95-108.

Bush, B. A. (1999). Major life events as risk factors for post-stroke depression. *Brain Injury, 13*(2), 131-137.

Centers for Disease Control. (1999). *Traumatic brain injury in the United States: A report to Congress.* Atlanta, GA: U.S. Department of Health and Human Services, National Center for Injury Prevention and Control.

Cohen, J. (1992). A power primer. *Psychological Bulletin, 112*(1), 155-159.

Cohen, N., Coyne, J., & Duvall, J. (1993). Adopted and biological children in the clinic: Family, parental and child characteristics. *Journal of Child Psychology and Psychiatry, 34*(4), 545-562.

Cohen, S., Kamarck, T., & Mermelstein, R. (1983). A global measure of perceived stress. *Journal of Health and Social Behavior, 24,* 385-396.

Cohen, S., Kessler, R., & Gordon, L. (Eds.). (1995). *Measuring stress: A guide for health and social scientists* (1st ed., Vol. 1). New York: Oxford University Press.

Davidson, R., Lewis, D., Alloy, L., Amaral, D., Bush, G., Cohen, J., et al. (2002). Neural and behavioral substrates of mood and mood regulation. *Biological Psychiatry, 52,* 478-502.

Dikmen, S., & Levin, H. (1993). Methodological issues in the study of mild head injury. *Journal of Head Trauma Rehabilitation, 8*(3), 30-37.

Fann, J., Katon, W., Uomoto, J., & Esselman, P. (1995). Psychiatric disorders and functional disability in outpatients with traumatic brain injuries. *American Journal of Psychiatry, 152*(10), 1493-1499.

Fann, J., Uomoto, J., & Katon, W. (2001). Cognitive improvement with treatment of depression following mild traumatic brain injury. *Psychosomatics, 42*(1), 48-54.

Fenton, G., McClelland, R., Montgomery, A., MacFlynn, G., & Rutherford, W. (1993). The postconcussional syndrome: Social antecedents and psychological sequelae. *British Journal of Psychiatry, 162,* 493-497.

Gold, P., Goodwin, F., & Chrousos, G. (1988). Clinical and biochemical manifestations of depression: Relationship to the neurobiology of stress (Part 2). *New England Journal of Medicine, 319*(2), 413-420.

Goldstein, L. (2003). Neuropharmacology of TBI-induced plasticity. *Brain Injury, 17*(8), 685-694.

Hellawell, D., Taylor, R., & Pentland, B. (1999). Cognitive and psychosocial outcome following moderate or severe traumatic brain injury. *Brain Injury, 13*(7), 489-504.

Holsinger, T., Steffens, D., Phillips, C., Helms, M., Havlik, R., Breitner, J., et al. (2002). Head injury in early adulthood and the lifetime risk of depression. *Archives in General Psychiatry, 59*(1), 17-22.

Jorge, R., Robinson, R., Arndt, S., Forrester, A., Geisler, F., & Starkstein, S. (1993). Comparison between acute and delayed onset depression following traumatic brain injury. *Journal of Neuropsychiatry, 5*(1), 43-49.

Jorge, R., Robinson, R., Arndt, S., Starkstein, S., Forrester, A., & Geisler, F. (1993). Depression following traumatic brain injury: A 1-year longitudinal study. *Journal of Affective Disorders, 27,* 233-243.

Kendall, E., & Terry, D. J. (1996). Psychosocial adjustment following closed head injury: A model for understanding individual differences and predicting outcomes. *Neuropsychological Rehabilitation, 6*(2), 101-132.

Kessler, R., & Magee, W. (1993). Childhood adversities and adult depression: Basic patterns of association in a US national survey. *Psychological Medicine,* 679-690.

Kinsella, G., Moran, C., Ford, B., & Ponsford, J. (1988). Emotional disorder and its assessment within the severe head injured population. *Psychological Medicine, 18,* 57-63.

Kreutzer, J., Marwitz, J., Seel, R., & Serio, C. (1996). Validation of a neurobehavioral functioning inventory for adults with traumatic brain injury. *Archives of Physical Medical Rehabilitation, 77*(2), 116-124.

Kreutzer, J., Seel, R., & Gourley, E. (2001). The prevalence and symptom rates of depression after traumatic brain injury: A comprehensive examination. *Brain Injury, 15*(7), 563-576.

Kreutzer, J., Seel, R., & Marwitz, J. (1999). *Neurobehavioral Functioning Inventory* (tm) (1st ed.). San Antonio, TX: Harcourt Brace.

Kupfer, D. J., & Detre, T. P. (1974). *K.D.S.: A Modern Mental Health Charting System* (1st ed., Vol. 1). Pittsburgh, PA: University of Pittsburgh Press.

Ladd, C., Owens, M., & Nemeroff, C. (1996). Persistent changes in corticotropin-releasing factor neuronal systems induced by maternal deprivation. *Endocrinology, 137*(4), 1212-1218.

Levin, H., Williams, D., Eisenberg, H., High, W., & Guinto, F. (1992). Serial MRI and neurobehavioral findings after mild to moderate closed head injury. *Journal of Neurology, Neurosurgery, and Psychiatry, 55,* 255-262.

Levin, H. S., Brown, S. A., Song, J., McCauley, S., Boake, C., Constant, C., et al. (2001). Depression and posttraumatic stress disorder at three months after mild-to-moderate traumatic brain injury. *Journal of Clinical and Experimental Neuropsychology, 23*(6), 754-769.

Liu, D., Diorio, J., Tannenbaum, B., Caldji, C., Francis, D., & Freedman, A. (1997, September 12). Maternal care, hippocampal glucocorticoid receptors, and hypothalamic-pituitary-adrenal responses to stress. *Science, 277,* 1659-1662.

Malia, K., Powell, G., & Torode, S. (1995). Coping and psychosocial function after brain injury. *Brain Injury, 9*(6), 607-618.

Martelli, M., Zasler, N., & MacMillan, P. (1998). Mediating the relationship between injury, impairment and disability: A vulnerability, stress and coping model of adaptation following brain injury. *NeuroRehabilitation, 11,* 51-66.

McCauley, S., Boake, C., Levin, H. S., Contant, C., & Song, J. (2001). Postconcussional disorder following mild to moderate traumatic brain injury: Anxiety, depression and social support as risk factors and comorbidities. *Journal of Clinical and Experimental Neuropsychology, 23*(6), 792-808.

McCleary, C., Satz, P., Forney, D., Light, R., Zaucha, K., Asarnow, R., et al. (1998). Depression after traumatic brain injury as a function of Glasgow Outcome Score. *Journal of Clinical and Experimental Neuropsychology, 20*(2), 270-279.

McEwen, B. (2002). *The end of stress as we know it* (1st ed.). Washington, DC: Joseph Henry Press.

Mooney, G., & Speed, J. (2001). The association between mild traumatic brain injury and psychiatric conditions. *Brain Injury, 10*(3), 492-501.

Nemeroff, C. (1998). The neurobiology of depression. *Scientific American, 6,* 42-49.

Nolen-Hoeksema, S. (1987). Sex differences in unipolar depression: Evidence and theory. *Psychological Bulletin, 101,* 259-282.

Ownsworth, T., & Oei, T. (1998). Depression after traumatic brain injury: Conceptualization and treatment considerations. *Brain Injury, 12*(9), 735-751.

Panel of the National Institutes of Health. (1999). Rehabilitation of persons with traumatic brain injury: NIH consensus statement. *Journal of the American Medical Association, 282,* 974-983.

Post, R. (1992). Transduction of psychosocial stress into the neurobiology of recurrent affective disorder. *American Journal of Psychiatry, 149*(8), 999-1009.

Raskin, S. (1997). The relationship between sexual abuse and mild traumatic brain injury. *Brain Injury, 11*(8), 587-603.

Rimel, R., Giordani, B., Barth, J., Boll, T., & Jane, J. (1981). Disability caused by minor head injury. *Neurosurgery, 9*(3), 221-228.

Satz, P., Forney, D., Zaucha, K., Asarnow, R., Light, R., McCleary, C., et al. (1998). Depression, cognition, and functional correlates of recovery outcome after traumatic brain injury. *Brain Injury, 12*(7), 537-553.

Schaeffer, M., & Baum, A. (1984). Adrenal cortical response to stress at Three Mile Island. *Psychosomatic Medicine, 46*(3), 227-236.

Seel, R., Kreutzer, J., Rosenthal, M., Hammond, F., Corrigan, J., & Black, K. (2003). Depression after traumatic brain injury: A National Institute on disability and rehabilitation model system research investigation. *Archives Physical Medicine Rehabilitation, 84*(2), 177-184.

Sliwinski, M., Gordon, W., & Bogdany, A. (1998). The Beck Depression Inventory: Is it a suitable measure of depression for individuals with traumatic brain injury. *Journal of Head Injury Rehabilitation, 13*(4), 40-46.

Wells, K., Stewart, A., Hays, R., Burnam, A., Rogers, W., Daniels, M., et al. (1989). The functioning and well being of depressed patients. *Journal of the American Medical Association, 262*(7), 914-919.

Williams, R. A., Hagerty, B. M., Cimprich, B., Therrien, B., Bay, E., & Oe, H. (2000). Changes in directed attention and short-term memory in depression. *Journal of Psychiatric Research, 34,* 227-238.

Young, E., Abelson, J., Curtis, G., & Nesse, R. (1997). Childhood adversity and vulnerability to mood and anxiety disorders. *Depression and Anxiety, 5,* 66-72.

8

The Relationship Between Maternal and Child Mental Health in Mexican Immigrant Families

Diane B. McNaughton
Julia Muennich Cowell
Deborah Gross
Louis Fogg
Sarah H. Ailey

Depression, which is estimated to occur in 9.5% of the U.S. population, is 1 of the 10 leading causes of disability in the United States (National Institute of Mental Health [NIMH], 2001). Persons with depression may experience a range of symptoms including lack of energy, social withdrawal, difficulty concentrating, and feelings of hopelessness or worthlessness (Kramlinger, 2001). Depression is also a primary risk factor for suicide (Kessler, Borges & Walters, 1999; Lopez & Katz, 2001; NIMH, 2001). There is evidence that Mexican immigrants, particularly Mexican immigrant women, report depressive symptoms at rates above the national average (U.S. Department of Health and Human Services, 2001), with rates ranging from 20% to 64% of the population (Alderete, Vega, Kolody, & Aguilar-Gaxiola, 1999; Codina & Montalvo, 1994; Finch, Kolody, & Vega, 2000; Hovey, 2000; Munet-Vilaro, Folkman, & Gregorich, 1999; Salgado de Snyder, Cervantes, & Padilla, 1990). This heightened depression rate is noteworthy given that Mexicans comprise the largest immigrant population in the United States (U.S. Government, n.d.).

In accordance with Healthy People 2010 objectives ("Healthy People 2010," 2000), mental health promotion is a national health priority. Therefore, it is essential that health care providers gain a complete understanding of the factors associated with depression in Mexican immigrant women as a foundation for developing health promotion programs for this population. The goal of this study is to identify variables associated with poorer mental health in Mexican immigrant women that can be used to design a nursing intervention for promoting mental health in Mexican immigrant families.

Several studies have previously identified factors associated with depression among Mexican immigrants. These include lower educational achievement (Heilemann, Lee, & Kury, 2002; Munet-Vilaro et al., 1999; Salgado de Snyder et al., 1990), lower socioeconomic status (Codina & Montalvo, 1994; Cueller & Roberts, 1997; Finch et al., 2000; Hovey, 2000), female gender (Codina & Montalvo, 1994; Munet-Vilaro et al., 1999; Salgado de Snyder et al., 1990; Vega, Warheit, Buhl-Aoth, & Meinhardt, 1984), and marital separation (Vega, Kolody, & Valle, 1986). Other studies have shown that quality of family and social relationships are important predictors of depression in Mexican immigrant women. For example, Hovey (2000) found a positive relationship between family dysfunction and women's depressive symptoms. In addition, the perceived effectiveness of the women's social support network was negatively associated with depressive symptoms and suicidal ideation. Vega and colleagues (Vega, Kolody, & Valle, 1986; Vega, Kolody, Valle, & Hough, 1986) found that women who had the support of a confidant reported fewer depressive symptoms. Taken together, these results indicate that women with fewer economic and social resources and less support are at higher risk for depression.

Many authors suggest that the causes of depression in Mexican immigrants may be due to the stress of acculturation (Alderete et al., 1999; Heilemann et al., 2002; Hovey, 2000; Hovey & King, 1997; Munet-Vilaro et al., 1999; Salgado de Snyder, 1987; Vega, Kolody, Valle, & Hough 1986). However, the results of these studies have been conflicting. For example, Alderete and associates (1999) reported more depressive symptoms among more acculturated women. In contrast, Vega, Kolody, Valle, and Hough (1986) found higher depression scores among Mexican immigrants living in the United States less than 6 years. Two other studies found no relationship between acculturation and mental health (Cuellar & Roberts, 1997; Masten, Penland, & Nayani, 1994). These conflicting results are difficult to interpret, in part because different measures to assess acculturation have been used in different studies. To date, the relationship between acculturation and depression remains unclear.

It is possible that the relationship between acculturation and depression may be a function of stress and family conflict arising from immigration rather than solely from the process of adapting to a new culture. For example, Salgado de Snyder (1987) found a significant relationship between acculturative stress and depression among Mexican immigrant married women in California. However, women who reported greater support from their spouses in the form of communication and intimacy reported fewer depressive symptoms. In another study, Salgado de Snyder and colleagues (1990) examined depressive symptoms and stress in 264 Mexican and Central American immigrants and found that for both cultural groups, women experienced a high degree of cultural/family conflict and marital stress. Aranda and associates (2001) also found that depression among low-income Mexican immigrant women was related to the quality of family and marital relationships. These data suggest that within the context of becoming acculturated, stress and family relationships play an important role in predicting Mexican immigrant women's mental health.

Although the research points to the importance of family relationships, relatively little work has been done on depression and the parent-child relationship among Mexican immigrant females. de Leon Siantz (1990) reported higher depression scores among Mexican American mothers who were migrant farmworkers and who had difficulty securing childcare. Although the research on maternal depression in the general population points to a consistent relationship between depression and poor outcomes in children (Gross, Conrad, Fogg, Willis, & Garvey, 1995; Petterson & Albers, 2001), little is known about the children of Mexican immigrant mothers with elevated depressive symptoms. Of particular interest is the effect of the mother's stress and depression on her children's mental health and well-being.

In summary, Mexican immigrant women suffer from more depressive symptoms than men and women in the general population, and their depression tends to be associated with the quality of the support they receive from family members. However, relatively little is known about the association between maternal and child mental health and what aspects of the family's functional quality are related to depressive symptoms. Further study is also needed on the role of acculturation and stress in understanding the high rate of depression in Mexican immigrant women. The purposes of this study are to: (a) describe mental health symptoms in a sample of Mexican immigrant mothers; (b) examine the relationship between maternal and children mental health; and (c) describe the relationships among maternal and child mental health, family hardiness, family functioning, and acculturation. For the purposes of this study, maternal mental health is defined as the mother's self-reported levels of depression, anxiety, and stress. Children's mental health is defined as the child's self-reported levels of depression and stress.

METHODS

This study is a secondary data analysis from the Rush Mexican American Problem Solving Program (Rush MAPS; Cowell, Ailey, McNaughton, & Gross, 2002). The Rush MAPS program is a clinical trial of a nursing intervention designed to assist Mexican immigrant mothers and their fourth and fifth grade children in maintaining and promoting their mental health. The secondary data analysis is based on baseline data collected when participants entered the study.

Sample

Mothers and their fourth and fifth grade children were recruited from public elementary schools in Chicago. The elementary schools are located in two neighborhoods: One is primarily populated by Mexican immigrants and the other neighborhood is ethnically diverse. Schools in the ethnically diverse neighborhood reported more than 30 primary languages spoken by their students. School personnel and bilingual research staff recruited families through parent meetings, classroom visits, and snowballing procedures.

Procedures

Data were collected by bilingual school social workers or bilingual graduate students. Data collectors received 8 hours of training and also received a data collection manual. Mothers were paid $30 for the baseline data collection and children were given a small gift worth about $2. Women participating in the study signed informed consents printed in Spanish and English, and children signed an assent sheet at the first data collection home visit. The initial data collection visit took about 90 minutes and included private interviews with mothers and children. Data collectors read the surveys with the mothers and children to account for literacy deficits.

Measures

Most of the research measures were available in Spanish. Instruments that were not available in Spanish were translated to Spanish and back translated (Cowell, McNaughton, & Ailey, 2000). A committee review at each step resolved disagreements and assured conceptual equivalence following the de-centering approach (Varrichio, 1997). For those instruments available in Spanish, a focus group of Mexican Americans with Spanish as their primary language reviewed translations to assure conceptual equivalence. Individual items were adjusted to reflect conceptual equivalence versus literal translations.

Mother's mental health was assessed using the Hopkins Symptom Checklist (HSC; Derogatis, Lipman, Rickels, Uhlenhuth, & Covi, 1974), a 25-item, self-rated measure of mental health consisting of two subscales, anxiety and depression. Scores on the HSC can range from 1 to 4 (scores are calculated by summing the item responses and dividing by the number of items answered). Persons with scores of 1.75 or higher are considered at increased risk and were referred for further evaluation. The alpha reliabilities for the anxiety and depression subscales were .89 and .91, respectively, indicating that both subscales are internally consistent. However, the anxiety and depression subscale scores were highly correlated ($r = .72$), which suggests that the two subscales are tapping a similar construct of maternal mental health. Therefore, a total HSC score will be used to estimate maternal depression and anxiety rather than analyzing each subscale separately. Alpha reliability for the total HSC in this sample was .94. The validity of the HSC with Mexican immigrant women was demonstrated through statistically significant correlations of the theoretically hypothesized relationships including family function and child depression (Cowell et al., 2000).

Mother's stress was measured using the Everyday Stress Index (ESI) developed by Hall (1983). The ESI measures the extent to which the parent is "bothered by" financial concerns, employment problems, parenting concerns, family responsibilities, and interpersonal conflicts. Items are scored on a range of 1 ("not at all bothered") to 4 ("bothered a great deal"). The validity of the ESI has been supported in previous studies by its significant associations with maternal depression, parenting self-efficacy, and children's behavior problems (Gross, Sambrook, & Fogg,

1999; Hall, 1990). To address stressors associated with child rearing, 10 additional items were added to the ESI (Adams-Wheeler & Gross, 1997). These items ask mothers the extent to which they are bothered by things such as "the amount of time you must spend away from your child," "your child's safety and well-being," "other children being a bad influence on your child," and "your child being too demanding of you and your time." Cronbach's alpha on these 30 stress items (20 from the ESI and the 10 additional items on child-related stressors) was .91. Item-to-total correlations for the 20 items from the ESI ranged from .37 to .56. The item-to-total correlations for the additional 10 items ranged from .37 to .61.

Family Functioning was measured using the Feetham Family Functioning Survey (FFFS; Roberts & Feetham, 1982). The FFFS assesses three primary areas of family function:

1. family relationships within the family and its subsystems,
2. division of labor, and
3. reciprocal relationships within the family and each individual family member.

The response set is designed in the Porter format (Porter, 1962, 1963a, 1963b), which captures the perceived magnitude, importance, and degree of need satisfaction. For each item, the informant indicates the degree to which the need is being satisfied in the family relationships, the degree to which the need should be satisfied in the family, and the importance of this need to the informant (Roberts & Feetham, 1982). A discrepancy score of the degree to which the need is being satisfied and the degree to which the need should be satisfied is also calculated. Higher discrepancy scores indicate poorer family functioning. Finally, an importance score was calculated to examine the individual's values and the relationship of their importance to the attainment of the function. Discrepancy and importance scores can be used to identify areas of perceived need and for nursing intervention. The validity of the FFFS with Mexican immigrant women was established in pilot work by a nominated group method. Specifically, mothers with known family dysfunction reported higher discrepancy scores indicating lower family function (Cowell et al., 2000). Cronbach's alpha for the instrument in this sample was .85.

Family hardiness was assessed using the Family Hardiness Index (FHI; McCubbin, McCubbin, & Thompson, 1986). Family hardiness refers to internal strengths and durability of the family unit and is characterized by a sense of control over life events. The FHI is a 20-item scale with three subscales: commitment, challenge, and control. The instrument is scored by summing the values of all responses (range of 0-3 possible for each item) with higher scores indicating greater family hardiness. McCubbin and colleagues (1986) reported validity studies of FHI by showing positive association with hardiness and other indicators of family strengths. The measures of family strength included family flexibility (FACES II), Family, Time and Routines, and Quality of Family Life. The correlations of these measures with FHI were all statistically significant. For this sample, Cronbach's alpha was .77, thus indicating adequate reliability.

Acculturation to the United States was measured using the Acculturation and Structural Assimilation Scale (ASAS; Hazuda, Stern, & Haffner, 1988). The ASAS includes five subscales of acculturation and two subscales of structural assimilation. Five of the original seven subscales were used for this study: adult proficiency in English (3 items), adult patterns of English usage (10 items), value placed on Mexican heritage (3 items), attitude toward traditional family structure (7 items), and adult interaction with mainstream society (3 items). Higher scores indicate increased assimilation to American culture. Construct validity of the instrument was reported by Hazuda, Stern, and Haffner (1988). Cronbach's alpha for this study was .86.

Children's depression was assessed using the Children's Depression Inventory (CDI; Kovacs, 1992), a 27-item survey based on the Beck Depression Inventory (Kovacs, 1985). The CDI was developed for use with children aged 8 to 13 years (Saylor, Finch, Spirito, & Bennett, 1984). Scores for items range from 0 (no report of this symptom) to 2 (more severe experience of this symptom). Total scores can range from 0 to 54 with higher scores indicating more depressive symptoms. In this study, based on the cutoff score recommended by Kovacs (1992) for children at heightened risk, children with scores of 12 or higher were referred for further evaluation. Validity of the CDI was established in pilot work by nominated group method with higher scores among children with reported depressed affect (Cowell et al., 2000). Cronbach's alpha for CDI in this sample was .79, indicating adequate reliability.

Child stress was measured using the Child Stress Index (CSI; Attar, Guerra, & Tolan, 1994). The CSI contains 16 items that assess the domains of Circumscribed Events (such as death of a close family member or friend, hospitalization of a family member, destruction of personal property due to disaster or theft), Life Transitions (such as marriage in family, new baby, change of school or home), and Exposure to Violence (need to hide from shootings, need to stay indoors because of gangs or drugs in neighborhood). Two CSI items related to observed violence or death of someone close were omitted for redundancy, yielding a total score range of 0 to 14, with higher scores indicating greater child stress. Children complete the index by indicating if they have experienced any of the stressful events listed. Construct validity for the measure is reported by Attar and associates (1994). Cronbach's alpha for this sample was .66.

Analysis

Descriptive and correlational analyses were conducted for all maternal and child study variables. In addition, children's data were analyzed separately by gender to determine if boys' and girls' mental health symptoms were differentially related to mothers' mental health. Finally, multiple regression analyses were conducted to examine whether child self-report measures (depression and stress) or mother's self-report measures (acculturation, family hardiness, stress) are stronger predictors of maternal mental health.

RESULTS

The sample consisted of 182 women and their 4th- and 5th-grade children. All of the women were born in Mexico and currently residing in the US. Length of time living in the US ranged from 6 months to 34 years (*M* = 12.2 years, *SD* = 7.3 years). The age of the mothers ranged from 23 to 65 years (*M* = 35.6 years, *SD* = 6.9 years). The mean age of the children was 10.2 years (SD = .82). There were 84 boys and 98 girls in the sample.

Most (82.9%) of the mothers were married or living with a partner and most (78.6%) claimed total household incomes less than $500/week or $27,000 per year. Less than half of the mothers (48%) had received education beyond primary school. Forty-one percent of the mothers reported working full or part time outside of their homes.

Means and standard deviations for all study variables are shown in Table 8.1. Mean acculturation scores were 40.06 (*SD* = 11.7, range 23-90), a relatively low acculturation score that suggests a preference within this sample for Mexican cultural values. The mean maternal mental health score on the HSC was 1.65 (*SD* = 0.52) and 61 mothers (33.5%) exceeded the cut-point of 1.75 for referral for further evaluation. Four women (2%) expressed suicidal ideation. Three of these four women indicated that they thought about ending their lives "quite a bit" ("frequemente") and one woman expressed that she was extremely ("extremadament") bothered about thoughts related to ending her life. All of these women were immediately contacted and received further assessment and treatment.

The mean child depression score on the CDI was 9.53 (*SD* = 5.8, range = 0-25). There were no differences in depression scores by gender (*M* for girls = 9.55, *SD* = 6.0; *M* for boys = 9.52, *SD* = 5.6). Thirty-one percent (*n* = 56) of the children received a CDI score above the cutoff for referral for further evaluation for depression. Of the children who exceeded the CDI cutoff score for depression, 51% (*n* = 31) had a mother whose mental health score also exceeded the standardized cutoff score.

TABLE 8.1. Means, Standard Deviations, and Ranges for Maternal, Child, and Family Health and Acculturation Scores (*n* = 182)

Variable	Score Range	*M*	*SD*
Maternal Depression/Anxiety	1.00-3.48	1.65	0.52
Family Functioning	0.0-79.0	29.00	18.25
Family Hardiness	15.0-59.0	42.18	7.81
Maternal Stress	35.0-117.0	71.52	17.44
Acculturation	23.0-90.0	40.06	11.67
Child Depression	0.0-25.0	9.53	5.76
Child Stress	0.0-10.0	3.92	2.53

The relationships among the maternal mental health, family functioning discrepancy scores, acculturation, and children's mental health are presented in Table 8.2. Maternal depression and anxiety as measured by the HSC was highly correlated with family functioning ($r = .57, p < .001$) and with mother's stress levels ($r = .45, p < .001$). There was a moderate correlation between maternal depression and anxiety and family hardiness ($r = -.35, p < .001$). However, maternal depression and anxiety were unrelated to acculturation as measured by the ASAS ($r = .07, p = ns$). When acculturation was reexamined using (a) number of years mother lived in the US and (b) the English language acquisition subscale from the ASAS, associations between these measures of acculturation and mothers' and children's mental health continued to be nonsignificant.

Children's stress and depression scores were not related to one another ($r = .10, p = ns$). However, both child mental health scores were significantly related to their mother's depression and anxiety ($r = .28, p < .001$ for child stress; $r = .22, p < .01$ for child depression). In addition, child mental health scores were significantly related to maternal stress ($r = .19, p < .05$ for child stress; $r = .25, p < .001$ for child depression). Finally, family functioning discrepancy scores were associated with child stress ($r = .30, p < .001$).

To examine whether the relationships among maternal and child mental health differed by child gender, the data were analyzed separately for boys and girls. The results of this analysis revealed that boys' depression scores were correlated with maternal reports of family functioning ($r = .23, p < .01$) and maternal stress ($r = .28, p < .01$) but unrelated to mothers' depression and anxiety ($r = .16, p = ns$). In contrast, girls' depression scores were correlated with maternal depression and anxiety ($r = .26, p < .01$) and maternal stress ($r = .23, p < .05$) but unrelated to family functioning ($r = .06, p = ns$). However, children's stress across genders was significantly related to maternal depression and anxiety ($r = .28, p < .05$ for boys, $r = .27$,

TABLE 8.2. Correlations Among Maternal, Child, and Family Health Variables and Acculturation (*n* = 182)

Variable	1	2	3	4	5	6	7
1. Maternal depression/anxiety	.94[a]						
2. Maternal stress	.45***	.91					
3. Family Functioning[b]	.57***	.41***	.85				
4. Family Hardiness	-.35***	-.10	-.18*	.77			
5. Acculturation	.07	.16*	.15*	.30**	.86		
6. Child depression	.22**	.25**	.14	-.12	.01	.79	
7. Child stress	.28**	.19**	.30**	.20	.07	.10	.66

Note. All 2-tailed tests.
[a]Scale reliabilities are presented along the diagonal.
[b]Higher scores indicate poorer family functioning.
*$p < .05$. **$p < .01$. ***$p < .001$.

$p < .05$ for girls) and poorer family functioning ($r = .29$, $p < .01$ for boys, $r = .31$, $p < .01$ for girls). These data indicate that poorer maternal mental health and family functioning are associated with greater stress in Mexican immigrant children (Table 8.3).

Two multiple regression analyses were conducted using mother's mental health (based on the HSC) as a dependent variable. The first examined the independent effects of child depression (CDI) and stress (CSI) on mothers' mental health followed by the mothers' self-reported estimates of acculturation (ASAS), stress (ESI revised), and family hardiness (FHI). Child stress and depression were significantly associated with maternal mental health ($\beta = .26$, $p < .01$ and $\beta = .18$, $p = .01$ respectively) and explained 11.3% of the variance. Adding family hardiness, maternal stress, and acculturation to this model increased the R^2 to 39% (with significant betas of -.40, $p = < .01$ for family hardiness; .32, $p = < .01$ for maternal stress; and .29, $p = < .01$ for child stress). In this model, acculturation and child depression were no longer significantly associated with maternal mental health. In particular, the CDI demonstrated the worst collinearity statistics associated with the analysis (tolerance = .93 and VIF = 1.08).

DISCUSSION

There are several important findings in this study. First, approximately one third of the mothers and children in this study are at heightened risk for mental health problems. Specifically, 33.5% of women in this study reported depression and anxiety symptoms at or above the designated cut-point for referral. For depression, this rate is comparable to that of Mexican immigrants in general but higher than the national average of 9.5% for Americans as reported by the NIMH (2003). Similarly, almost one third (31%) of the Mexican immigrant children in this sample scored in the depressed range on the CDI. Of particular importance is that of the children whose scores fell into the depressed range, 51% had a mother whose depression

TABLE 8.3. Relationship Between Maternal and Child Mental Health Variables by Child Gender (*n* = 182)

Variable	Boys' Depression	Boys' Stress	Girls' Depression	Girls' Stress
Maternal depression/anxiety	.16	.28**	.26**	.27**
Maternal stress	.28**	.19	.23*	.15
Family functioning[a]	.23*	.29**	.06	.31**
Family hardiness	-.14	.26*	-.08	.16
Acculturation	.06	.10	-.03	.04

Note. All 2-tailed tests.
[a]Higher scores indicate poorer family functioning.
$^{*}p < .05$. $^{**}p < .01$.

and anxiety score also exceeded the standardized cutoff. These findings suggest that (a) a large portion of Mexican immigrant mothers and children are in need of evaluation for mental health problems and (b) depressed children are likely to have mothers with mental health concerns as well.

For mothers in this study, depression and anxiety were most strongly correlated with their assessment of family functioning as measured by the perceived discrepancies between what the mothers wanted and what they felt they were receiving in their family relationships ($r = .57, p < .001$). These findings are consistent with those reported by others showing that women with greater family dysfunction, poorer marital relationships, and fewer social supports are at greater risk for mental health problems (Hovey, 2000; Jones, Beach, & Forehand, 2001; Vega, Kolody, & Valle, 1986). The finding is also congruent with Mexican cultural values of familialism, in which family (extended and nuclear) is central and provides support to individuals during times of stress (de Leon Siantz, 1994; Meleis, Douglas, Eribes, Shih, & Messias, 1996). It is logical that in a culture where family is an essential support system, that women who are unhappy with the way their families function may also have symptoms of anxiety and depression.

Family hardiness scores were inversely related to women's depressive symptoms ($r = -.35, p < .000$). McCubbin and colleagues (1986) describe family hardiness as a stress resistance and adaptation resource for families that acts as a buffer against the effects of stressors and demands, and facilitates family resiliency adjustment and adaptation over time. As would be expected, family hardiness scores in this study were inversely related to family functioning scores ($r = -.18$). While family hardiness may be an immutable characteristic, it could serve as an indicator for families or women needing support.

All of the mothers in this sample were born in Mexico. Yet acculturation was unrelated to maternal depression and anxiety. This finding held true regardless of the method used to estimate acculturation (i.e., the ASAS, years living in the US, or language preference). However, acculturation was weakly associated with greater stress ($r = .16$) and family dysfunction ($r = .15$). These results suggest that although acculturation does not lead to depression and anxiety in Mexican immigrant women, it may still create problems, particularly as the women enter the workforce and are expected to contribute financially to the family (Meleis et al., 1996; Munet-Vilaro et al., 1999). For example, 41% of the mothers in this sample were employed but almost half had little education beyond the primary grades, increasing the odds that jobs available to them are low prestige and low pay. Although most were married, most of the families claimed total household incomes well below the median. Given their educational and economic disadvantage, it is possible that many of these mothers may feel that their American dreams might not be fully realized. Mothers who are working and caring for children might also feel frustrated by their traditional Mexican marriages (Meleis et al., 1996).

Boys' and girls' mental health were differentially associated with their mothers' mental health. Specifically, mothers' anxiety and depression symptoms were correlated only with their daughters' depressive symptoms. In contrast, the boys' depressive symptoms were correlated with maternal stress and poorer family functioning. Nonetheless, both boys and girls reported greater stress when their mothers had elevated levels of depression and anxiety. These results suggest that boys and girls may experience negative effects from their mothers' mental health symptoms but in different ways. That is, girls may identify with their mothers' depression and anxiety while boys may react to the family conflict. It also suggests that the stressful issues that are affecting the mother are causing the children stress as well.

An important limitation of this study is that all of the data are correlational. Therefore, it is not possible to determine whether the mother's mental health problems caused her children to also experience mental health problems or vice versa. However, the findings do suggest that an intervention for promoting mental health in Mexican immigrant women must include the children given the overlap in symptomatology. The results also point to the importance of focusing on family functioning and the quality of the mother's relationships with other members of the family.

Implications for Research and Practice

The prevalence of mental health symptoms for both mothers and children in this study underscore the importance of screening for depression and anxiety in this population. Ideally, screening should be done during routine health care visits. However, access to health care for low-income families is limited (U.S. Surgeon General, 2003). School-based screening programs (for parents and children) would be an avenue for assessing a population that may not have access to regular health care. The benefit of using public schools is that they are accessible to all families regardless of income or immigration status. In addition, Mexican immigrant families have considered their local schools to be a trusted source of help (Cowell et al., 2000). School nurses, social workers, and psychologists could provide support in the form of either mental health promotion interventions or assisting families in finding community resources.

Because of the differences in boys' and girls' responses to their mother's mental health symptoms, individualized interventions for boys and girls might be considered. Researchers have reported differences in boys' and girls' responses when parents divorce, with boys exhibiting externalizing behaviors such as behavior disorders and problems in interpersonal relations at home and at school that are often sustained for several years (Heatherington, Stanley-Hagan, & Anderson, 1989). In contrast, girls' emotional and social disturbances related to divorce often dissipate in a shorter period of time (Heatherington et al., 1989).

This descriptive study examined one sample of Mexican immigrant women and their children. Fathers were not included. It is quite possible that they, too, are experiencing mental health problems that are affecting the rest of the family. Future research should incorporate Mexican immigrant fathers to assess their mental health needs and how they perceive their families.

REFERENCES

Adams-Wheeler, K., & Gross, D. A. (1997). *Societal stress: A model on parenting in a low income minority population.* Unpublished manuscript, Rush University College of Nursing, Chicago.

Alderete, E., Vega, W. A., Kolody, B., & Aguilar-Gaxiola, S. (1999). Depressive symptomatology: Prevalence and psychosocial risk factors among Mexican migrant farmworkers in California. *Journal of Community Psychology, 27*(4), 457-471.

Aranda, M. P., Castaneda, I., Lee, P., & Sobel, E. (2001). Stress, social support, and coping as predictors of depressive symptoms: Gender differences among Mexican Americans. *Social Work Research, 25*(1), 37-48.

Attar, B. K., Guerra, N. G., & Tolan, P. H. (1994). Neighborhood disadvantage, stressful life events, and adjustment in urban elementary school children. *Journal of Clinical Child Psychology, 23,* 391-400.

Codina, G. E., & Montalvo, F. F. (1994). Chicano phenotype and depression. *Hispanic Journal of Behavioral Science, 16*(3, Suppl. 7), 296-306.

Cowell, J. M., Ailey, S. H., McNaughton, D. B., & Gross, D. (2002, September). *Fears, experiences and mental health of Mexican American children.* Paper presented at the State of the Science Congress, Washington, DC.

Cowell, J. M., McNaughton, D. B., & Ailey, S. (2000). Development and evaluation of a Mexican immigrant family support program. *Journal of School Nursing, 16,* 4-11.

Cuellar, I., & Roberts, R. (1997). Relations of depression, acculturation, and socioeconomic status in a Latino sample. *Hispanic Journal of Behavioral Sciences, 19*(2), 230-238.

de Leon Siantz, M. L. (1990). Correlates of maternal depression among Mexican-American migrant farmworker mothers. *Journal of Child and Adolescent Psychiatric Mental Health Nursing, 3*(1), 9-13.

Derogatis, L. R., Lipman, R. S., Rickels, K., Uhlenhuth, E. H., & Covi, L. (1974). The Hopkins Symptom Checklist (HSCL): A self-report symptom inventory. *Behavioral Science, 19,* 1-5.

Finch, B. K., Kolody, B., & Vega, W. A. (2000). Perceived discrimination and depression among Mexican-origin adults in California. *Journal of Health and Social Behavior, 41,* 295-313.

Gross, D., Conrad, B., Fogg, L., Willis, L., & Garvey, C. (1995). A longitudinal study of maternal depression and preschool children's mental health. *Nursing Research, 44,* 96-101.

Gross, D., Sambrook, A., & Fogg, L. (1999). Behavior problems among young children in low-income urban day care centers. *Research in Nursing and Health, 22*(1), 15-25.

Hall, L. A. (1983). *Social supports, everyday stressors, and maternal mental health.* Unpublished doctoral dissertation, University of North Carolina, Chapel Hill.

Hall, L. A. (1990). Prevalence and correlates of depressive symptoms in mothers of young children. *Public Health Nursing, 7*(2), 71-79.

Hazuda, H., Stern, M., & Haffner, S. (1988). Acculturation and assimilation among Mexican Americans: Scales and population-based data. *Social Science Quarterly, 69,* 687-706.

Healthy People 2010. *Leading health indicators: Priorities for action.* Retrieved September 19, 2003, from http://www.healthypeople.gov/LHI/Priorities.htm

Heatherington, E. M., Stanley-Hagan, M., & Anderson, E. R. (1989). Marital transitions: A child's perspective. *American Psychologist, 44*(2), 303-312.

Heilemann, M. V., Lee, K. A., & Kury, F. S. (2002). Strengths and vulnerabilities of women of Mexican descent in relation to depressive symptoms. *Nursing Research, 51*(3), 175-182.

Hovey, J. D. (2000). Acculturative stress, depression, and suicidal ideation in Mexican immigrants. *Cultural Diversity and Ethnic Minority Psychology, 6*(2), 134-151.

Hovey, J. D., & King, C. A. (1997). Suicidality among acculturating Mexican Americans: Current knowledge and directions for research. *Suicide and Life-Threatening Behavior, 27*(1), 92-103.

Jones, D. J., Beach, S. R. H., & Forehand, R. (2001). Stress generation in intact community families: Depressive symptoms, perceived family relationship stress, and implications for adolescent adjustment. *Journal of Social and Personal Relationships, 18*(4), 443-462.

Kessler, R. C., Borges, G., & Walters, E. (1999). Prevalence of and risk factors for lifetime suicide attempts in the national comorbidity survey. *Archives of General Psychiatry, 57*(7), 617-626.

Kovacs, M. (1985). The children's depression inventory. *Psychopharmacology Bulletin, 21,* 995-998.

Kovacs, M. (1992). *Children's depression inventory: Manual.* North Tonawanda, NY: Multi-Health Systems.

Kramlinger, K. (Ed). (2001). *Mayo clinic on depression.* Rochester, MN: Mayo Clinic.

Lopez, A. G., & Katz, I. (2001). An introduction to Latinos in the United States. In A. G. Lopez and E. Carrillo (Eds.), *The Latino psychiatric patient* (pp. 3-17). Washington, DC: American Psychiatric Publishing.

Masten, W. G., Penland, E. A., & Nayani, E. J. (1994). Depression and acculturation in Mexican-American women. *Psychological Reports, 75,* 1499-1503.

McCubbin, M. A., McCubbin, H. I., & Thompson, A. I. (1986). Family hardiness index (FHI). In H. I. McCubbin, A. I. Thompson, & M. A. McCubbin (1996) (Eds.), *Family assessment: Resiliency, coping and adaptation—Inventories for research and practice* (pp. 239-305). Madison: University of Wisconsin System.

Meleis, A. I., Douglas, M. K., Eribes, C., Shih, F., & Messias, D. K. (1996). Employed Mexican women as mothers and partners: Valued, empowered and overloaded. *Journal of Advanced Nursing, 23,* 82-90.

Munet-Vilaro, F., Folkman, S., & Gregorich, S. (1999). Depressive symptomatology in three Latino groups. *Western Journal of Nursing Research, 21*(2), 209-224.

National Institute of Mental Health. (2001). *The numbers count.* Retrieved July 28, 2003, from http://www.nimh.nih.gov/publicat/numbers.cfm

Petterson, S. M., & Albers, A. B. (2001). Effects of poverty and maternal depression on early child development. *Child Development, 72*(6), 1794-1813.

Porter, L. W. (1962). Job attitudes in management: Part I. Perceived deficiencies in need fulfillment as a function of job level. *Journal of Applied Psychology, 46*(6), 375-384.

Porter, L. W. (1963a). Job attitudes in management: Part II. Perceived importance of needs as a function of job level. *Journal of Applied Psychology, 47*(2), 141-148.

Porter, L. W. (1963b). Job attitudes in management: Part III. Perceived deficiencies in need fulfillment as a function of line versus staff type of job. *Journal of Applied Psychology, 47*(4), 267-275.

Roberts, C. S., & Feetham, S. L. (1982). Assessing family functioning across three areas of relationships. *Nursing Research, 31*(4), 231-235.

Salgado de Snyder, V. N. (1987). Factors associated with acculturative stress and depressive symptomatology among married Mexican immigrant women. *Psychology of Women Quarterly, 11,* 475-488.

Salgado de Snyder, V. N., Cervantes, R. C., & Padilla, A. M. (1990). Gender and ethnic differences in psychosocial stress and generalized distress among Hispanics. *Sex Roles, 22*(7/8), 441-453.

Saylor, C. F., Finch, A. J., Spirito, A., & Bennett, B. (1984). The children's depression inventory: A systematic evaluation of psychometric properties. *Journal of Consulting and Clinical Psychology, 52*(6), 955-967.

U.S. Department of Health and Human Services. (2001). *Mental health: Culture, race, and ethnicity. A supplement to Mental Health: A report of the Surgeon General.* Washington, DC: Author.

U.S. Government. (n.d.). *Fiscal year 2002 yearbook of immigration statistics.* Retrieved August 29, 2003, from http://www.immigration.gov/graphics/shared/aboutus/statistics/IMM02yrbk/IMM2002list.htm

U.S. Surgeon General. (2003). *Culture, race and ethnicity. A supplement to mental health: A report of the Surgeon General.* Retrieved April 15, 2003, from http://www.surgeongeneral.gov/library/mentalhealth/cre/fact3.asp

Varricchio, C. (1997). Measurement issues concerning linguistic translations. In M. Frank-Stromber & J. J. Olson (Eds.), *Instruments for clinical health-care research* (2nd ed., pp. 54-58). Boston: Jones & Bartlett.

Vega, W. A., Kolody, B., Valle, R., & Hough, R. (1986). Depressive symptoms and their correlates among immigrant Mexican women in the United States. *Social Science and Medicine, 22*(6), 645-652.

Vega, W. A., Kolody, B., & Valle, J. R. (1986). The relationship of marital status, confidant support, and depression among Mexican immigrant women. *Journal of Marriage and the Family, 48,* 597-605.

Vega, W., Warheit, G., Buhl-Auth, J., & Meinhardt, K. (1984). The prevalence of depressive symptoms among Mexican Americans and Anglos. *American Journal of Epidemiology, 120*(4), 592-607.

Acknowledgment. This study is funded by NINR RO1 NRO5008-01A1.

9

Predictors of Depression in Thai Women

Sopin Sangon

Depression is one of the major mental health problems of the present time (McGrath, Keita, Strickland, & Russo, 1990). In the year 2020, depression is expected to be the second cause of morbidity and mortality for the world population (Murray & Lopaz, 1996). However, most striking about depression is its predominance in women (Nolen-Hoeksema, 1987, 1990; Weissman & Olfson, 1995). A large body of evidence indicates that women suffer both depressive affect and clinical depression more than men (Blazer, Kessler, McGonagle, & Swartz, 1994; Nolen-Hoeksema, 1987, 1990).

In Thailand, depression is also expected to be one of the major mental health problems in the near future. Recently, Thailand has experienced a severe economic crisis. During this crisis, the number of depressed patients increased rapidly. In 1997, the Ministry of Public Health of Thailand reported that the prevalence of depression in the Thai population was about 10% (Mental Health Department, 1997). Although there is no empirical evidence about the predominance of women experiencing depression in Thailand, rapid social and economic changes may have an impact on women's lives, in terms of roles and status.

These changes may create a situation where women's traditional roles no longer fit their current lives. There tends to be a negative relationship between a nation's industrialization process, including socioeconomic development and modernization, and the economic, social, and psychological development of women (Yoddumnern-Attig, Richer, Soonthorndhada, Sethaput, & Pramualratana, 1992). Being a woman and confronting great changes in social and economic conditions put Thai women at risk for developing depression, yet most available literature about depression in Thailand is focused on children and adolescents or the elderly. Because women assume important roles and make great contributions to the country, knowledge that enhances understanding depression in Thai women is important to guide mental health care.

There are a number of compelling reasons for conducting research on depression in Thai women; these include: (a) there is very little research about depression in Thai women; (b) evidence from the United States and other countries confirms that women are more likely to develop depression than men; (c) Thai women are at risk for developing depression because of their double jeopardy of being women and at a time when Thailand is experiencing social and economic transformation and severe economic problems; and (d) although some research has been conducted to understand the development and risk factors of depression in women in the West, study results were based on White or African American subjects. It is possible that women from different socioeconomic and cultural backgrounds may demonstrate different relationships among risk factors for depression or that other factors may be more important. Thus, the purpose of this study was to examine the predictors or risk factors of depression in Thai women.

The conceptual model of this study was developed by the author and was based on the literature about theories of depression, depression in women, and some observation and reports about women in current Thai society. There are three groups of variables in the model, including:

1. predisposing factors including family history of depression, loss of mother before aged 11, and previous history of depression;
2. stressors; and
3. psychosocial factors including social support and sense of belonging.

Most of the stressors included in this study were selected based on the reports and observation of women in current Thai society. Stressors that Thai women are more likely to experience are stressful life events, role strain, interpersonal conflict, and parental role strain.

The specific aims for this study were to: (a) describe the predictive value of family history of depression; early loss of mother before age 11; previous history of depression; stressors including stressful life events, role strains, interpersonal conflict, and parental role strain; social support; and sense of belonging on clinical depression in women in Thailand; and (b) examine the effects of family history of depression; early loss of mother before age 11; previous history of depression; stressors including stressful life events, role strains, interpersonal conflict, and parental role strain; social support; and sense of belonging on severity of depression in women in Thailand.

Figure 9.1 presents the proposed model for selected risk factors and their effects on depression in Thai women. The following nine hypotheses were tested in this study:

1. Depressed women will be more likely to have a family history of depression and past history of loss of mother before age 11 than nondepressed women.
2. Depressed women will have more stressful life events, higher perceived stress, higher role strain, higher interpersonal conflict, and higher parental role strain than nondepressed women.
3. Depressed women will have lower social support and lower sense of belonging than nondepressed women.
4. Predisposing factors (family history of depression and past history of loss of mother before age 11) will have direct effects on severity of depression.
5. Stressors (stressful life events, perceived stress, role strains, interpersonal conflict, and parental role strain) will have direct effects on the severity of depression.

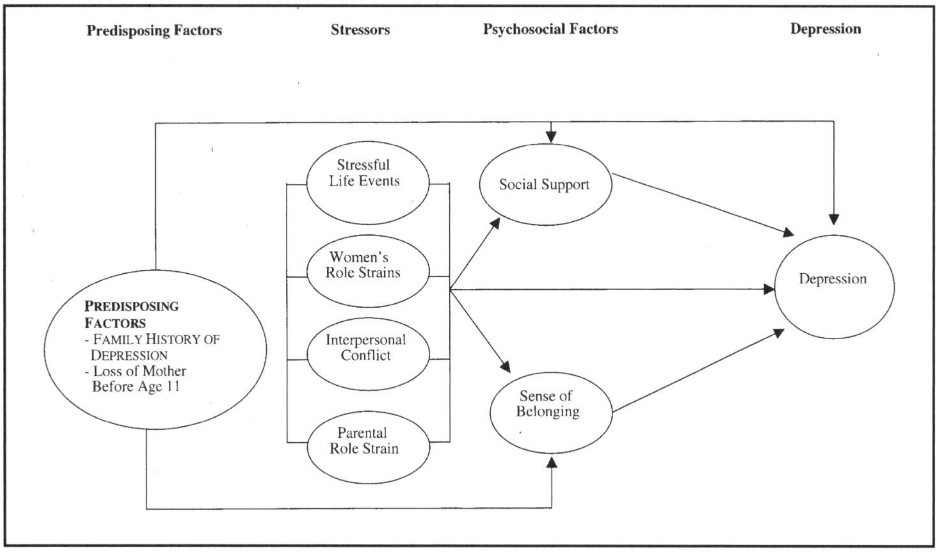

Figure 9.1. The proposed model predicting the effect of predisposing factors, stressor variables, and psychosocial factors on depression.

6. Psychosocial factors (social support and sense of belonging) will have direct effects on severity of depression.
7. Stressors (stressful life events, perceived stress, role strains, interpersonal conflict, and parental role strain) will mediate the effects of predisposing factors (family history of depression and past history of loss of mother before age 11) on severity of depression.
8. Psychosocial factors (social support and sense of belonging) will mediate the effects of predisposing factors (family history of depression and past history of loss of mother before age 11) on severity of depression.
9. Psychosocial factors (social support and sense of belonging) will mediate the effects of stressors (stressful life events, perceived stress, role strains, interpersonal conflict, and parental role strain) on severity of depression.

LITERATURE REVIEW

Depression

Depression has been recognized as a psychiatric illness since 1500 B.C. (Stuart, 1995) and viewed as a pervasive health care problem for decades. The problem raised in research studies on depression is to what extent the periods of depressive symptoms that do not meet criteria for a major depression as shown in DSM-IV differ from major depression (Nolen-Hoeksema, 1995). Yet the question has not been answered (Nolen-Hoeksema, 1995). However, it was discovered that persons with depressive symptoms were 4.4 times more likely to develop a first onset major depression over 1 year (Horwath, Johmson, Klerman, & Weissman, 1994). This result revealed the clinical significance of depressive symptoms, even if they do not meet the criteria for major depression (Horwath et al., 1994; Nolen-Hoeksema, 1995). In addition, depressive symptoms are found to be associated with decreased functioning in occupational, school, and social settings, as well as a diminished sense of well-being, and more disability (Horwath et al., 1994; Nolen-Hoeksema, 1995). Therefore, these milder forms of depression should not be ignored (Nolen-Hoeksema, 1995). To date, several theories have emerged in order to explain and understand depression. Biological explanations involve genetic transmission, neurotransmission, and neuroendocrinology. Psychological explanations include psychoanalytic, behavioral, cognitive, and self-in-relation theory, and the learned helplessness model. Social explanations include social role theory and the interpersonal relations model.

Family History of Depression

Family history of depression is defined as a person's information concerning the presence of depressed persons in his/her family (Zauszniewski, 1994). There is substantial evidence to support the risk of developing depression if a person has a family history of depression. This family lineage may occur genetically or through environmental influences and interpersonal relationships that generate stress, or both.

Having a depressed person in the family can have a significant impact on the other members in the family. There may be dysfunction such as "family interactions, parent-child relationship, communications, ability of problem-solving, and ability to show love and affection" in families of depressed persons (Zauszniewski, 1994, p. 16). Children may learn the emotions and behaviors of the depressed parents and use them when they confront stressful life events, thus ending up with depression (Zauszniewski, 1994).

Early Loss of Mother Before Age 11

Early loss of mother before age 11 is defined as a person's past experience of loss of mother by death or separation before age 11 (Brown & Harris, 1978). Brown and Harris found that only loss of mother before age 11 had a significant role on the development of depression. Based on Freud's theories, the early separation from parents can lead to disappointment and traumatic experiences in children. Later in life the trauma experiences can reactivate depressive conditions. Also, Brown and Harris found that childhood loss of mother can lead to a distinct life path which increases risk for experiencing stressful life events or chronic stress such as premarital pregnancy and poverty (Brown & Harris, 1978).

Stressful Life Events

Literature on depression has indicated that depression is often preceded by stressful life events (Brown, Bifulco, & Harris, 1987; Brown & Harris, 1978; Kendler, Karkowski, & Prescott, 1999; Kendler, Kessler, Neale, Health, & Eaves, 1993;

Lewinsohn & Hoberman, 1988; Monroe, Connell, Bromet, & Steiner, 1986). Stressful life events such as losing a job and loss of a loved one are important stressors, capable of producing depression (Brown & Harris, 1978). Monroe and colleagues (1986) found that an increased incidence of life events was related to an increased likelihood of subsequent depressive symptoms in married women. In addition, Kendler and associates (1993) provide strong evidence for the importance of stressful life events in the etiology of depression in women.

Role Strain

Role strain develops when a person occupying multiple roles experiences either role conflict or role overload (Stuart, 1981; Tiedje, 1987). Role conflict occurs when people struggle to manage the overwhelming, simultaneous, and inconsistent demands related to their total role sets (Tiedje, 1987). Role overload involves multiple roles that are probably too complex, competing for time as a scare resource (Tiedje, 1987). Role strain is viewed as constant stress arising out of a person's everyday social roles (Stuart, 1981). Women are thought to be more likely to experience role strain from their three major roles including employment, marriage, and motherhood. It is believed that the frustrations and conflicts arising from these demands may contribute to the development of depression in women (Aneshensel, Frerichs, & Clark, 1981; Cleary & Mechanic, 1983; Lennon & Rosenfield, 1992).

Interpersonal Conflict

Interpersonal conflict is defined as "the misunderstanding of a person, or the negative affect or tension directed at a person, from people considered to be significant to the person" (Abramis, 1985, p. 9). The quality of close relationships is an important factor associated with depressive symptoms in women.

Marital problems are also related to depressive symptoms (Coyne, Burchill, & Stiles, 1991). Paykel and colleagues (1969) found that depressed women reported arguments with husbands as the most frequent stressor prior to their onset of depression. In addition, Coyne and Downey (1991) reported that negative aspects of relationships like interpersonal conflict had stronger relationships with depression than positive aspects. In addition, in a society such as Thailand where the value of respecting others, especially older persons, family members, cousins, and significant others, is very high, it is logical to expect that interpersonal relationships produce stress in Thai people. Therefore, hypothesizing that interpersonal conflict will predict depressive symptoms in Thai women is appropriate.

Parental Role Strain

Women, as mothers, play an important role in raising children, providing basic needs, and providing important information about social values and norms. As a result of socioeconomic and cultural transformation in Thailand, Thai women are more likely to work outside their home in order to increase their household income. Working outside the home, women have found themselves confronted with less time to take care of their children. As a result children may receive less parental discipline, resulting in more problems such as drug use and gambling (Spielmann, 1994).

Women as parents, therefore, are under stress not only from role burdens but also from concerns about their children.

Social Support

Social support has been investigated extensively as having a positive impact on an individual's psychological well-being. In general, it is believed that social support enhances individuals' ability to effectively handle stress. A large body of empirical evidence has supported the notion that social support is an important factor in the individual psychological well-being in women (Aneshensel & Frerichs, 1982; Beeber, 1987; Boyce et al., 1998; Brugha, Bebbington, Stretch, MacCarthy, & Wykes, 1997; Kendler et al., 1993; Monroe et al., 1986; Paykel, 1994; Warren, 1995). Specifically, a lack of social support is associated with depressive symptoms (Paykel, 1994). Women with high levels of social support have a lower risk of developing depressive symptoms than women with no or low levels of social support (Warren, 1995).

Sense of Belonging

Sense of belonging is defined as "the experience of personal involvement in a system or environment so that persons feel themselves to be an integral part of that system or environment" (Hagerty, Lynch-Sauer, Patusky, Bouwsema, & Collier, 1992, p. 172). The person with a low level of psychological sense of belonging may be more likely to suffer from psychological, social, or physical problems and a weakened and unstable fundamental foundation for emotional and behavioral responses (Hagerty & Williams, 1999). On the other hand, a high level of psychological sense of belonging may support the person's psychological and social functioning (Hagerty, Williams, Coyne, & Early, 1996). Sense of belonging has not been widely investigated in relation to depression. Hagerty and Williams (1999) conducted a cross-sectional study to examine the effects of sense of belonging, social support, conflict, and loneliness on depression in depressed and nondepressed people and found that sense of belonging was a better predictor of depression than social support, conflict, and loneliness.

METHODS

Design

A cross-sectional comparative, correlational design was used to examine the effects of family history of depression; early loss of mother before age 11; previous history of depression; stressors including stressful life events, role strains, interpersonal conflict, and parental role strain; social support; and sense of belonging on depression in Thai women.

SUBJECTS

A convenience sample was used. Sample size was determined by power analysis for an alpha of .05, a power of .80, and a medium effect size. According to Cohen (1988), if using a *t* test with a medium effect size, a power of .80, and alpha of .05, a sample size of 128 subjects or 64 subjects per group was required. The final sample consisted of 142 women aged 19 to 68 years. The mean age of the women was 43.69 years ($SD = 10.80$). Participants who were or were not depressed were recruited from women at outpatient clinics at a major teaching hospital in Thailand.

General inclusion criteria were: Being a Thai woman aged 18 or older, and being able to read and write in the Thai language. Inclusion criteria for depressed women were having had a history of being diagnosed with major depression by a psychiatrist, and/or providing answers regarding having met the DSM-IV criteria for major depression either currently or previously on the short version of the Structured Clinical Interview for Depression (SCID). Inclusion criteria for nondepressed women were having no history of being diagnosed with major depression and/or having had negative answers regarding the DSM-IV criteria for major depression on the short version of the SCID at the time of interview.

PROCEDURES

Approval was obtained from the Institutional Review Board of the university where the author was enrolled as a graduate student; a similar process was followed in obtaining clearance and permissions from the teaching hospital in Thailand where data collection was to occur. The researcher then approached potential participants at the gynecological and psychiatric outpatient clinics at the data collection site located in Bangkok, the capital city of Thailand. A pilot study was conducted with women to test the usefulness of the instruments. Potential participants were approached and informed about the purpose of the study, and if they agreed to participate by oral consent, data collection was initiated. Data collection was conducted in a quiet room in each clinic. In the room, participants were informed again about the purpose of the study and the complete procedure for data collection. Due to a low literacy rate in Thailand, all participants were first interviewed using the questionnaires about personal information, the short version of the SCID and their past family history. Based on meeting study criteria from the first interview, participants were invited to participate in the study. At this point, participants were interviewed about the information from the seven questionnaires used in the study. The average time for completing the data collection procedure was approximately 1 hour to 1 1/2 hours for each participant. After completing the questionnaires, care was taken that participants were seen by their physicians at their expected time.

INSTRUMENTS

Some instruments were translated from English into the Thai language using the back translation technique and pilot tested prior to use in the study. The process of back translation technique was as follows: (a) the original English version of these instruments was translated into central Thai by the investigator, which is the dialect that all Thai people understand; (b) the Thai version of these instruments was translated back into English by independent translators who have skill in both languages; and (c) finally, the back-translated version of these instruments was compared by the investigator to the original version in order to identify discrepancies between the two instruments (Hulin, Drasgow, & Parsons, 1983).

Depression was measured by the Thai Depression Inventory (TDI) developed by Lotrakul and Sukanich (1999). It is a self-rating instrument with 20 items for measuring the severity of depression in Thai people. Each item of this 20-item inventory consists of four self-evaluative statements scored from 0 to 3 according to intensity. The items are summed to calculate a total depression score, with increasing scores indicating greater severity of depression (Lotrakul & Sukanich, 1999). The scale appears to have good validity. The internal consistency coefficients for the total scale of the TDI was 0.86. The internal consistency coefficient for a pilot study and the current study were 0.83 and 0.94 respectively.

Family history of depression was determined by asking participants a question about the presence or absence of depressive disorders in first-degree relatives such as parents, siblings, and grandparents.

Loss of mother before age 11 was determined by verbally asking questions regarding the age at which loss of mother had occurred and mechanisms through which the loss had taken place, such as death or separation.

Previous history of depression was assessed by the short version of SCID adapted from DSM-IV Structured Clinical Interview for Major Depression and used as a "yes" or "no" format. Using the SCID, participants were assessed for both current and previous episodes of depression.

Stressful life events was measured by the Perceived Stress Scale (PSS) and the Stress Event Checklist. The PSS was developed by Cohen, Kamarck, and Mermelstein (1983) and was designed to measure the extent to which situations in one's life are appraised as stressful in the last month. The PSS consists of 14 items on a 5-point Likert-type scale from "never" to "very often." The items are summed to calculate a total perceived stress score, with increasing scores indicating higher perceived stress. Cronbach's alpha for the PSS ranged from 0.84 to 0.86 (Cohen et al., 1983). The PSS was translated into Thai before being used in the study. Cronbach's alpha for a pilot study and the current study were 0.82 and 0.94 respectively. This scale was found to have adequate validity (Cohen et al., 1983).

The Stress Event Checklist was used to assess participants' experiences of negative life events. Events that are included in this checklist are negative events that have been found to correlate highly with depression (Brugha, Bebbington, Tennant, & Hurry, 1985). An index was formed by summing the number of major negative life events that occurred for the participants in the last 6 months from a list of such events. The range of possible scores for the index is 0 through 13, with higher scores indicating more negative life events experienced. The internal consistency for this instrument was not examined since the life events items included in this instrument are independent of each other. Before being used in the study, the Stress Event Checklist was translated into Thai. From a pilot study, the Stress Events Checklist was found to be clear and understandable for Thai women.

Women's role strain was measured by the Women's Role Strain Inventory (WRSI) and the Role Burden and Role Overload Questionnaire. Both instruments were translated into Thai prior to use with the subjects in the study. The WRSI was developed by Lengacher in 1993 based on Goode's theory of role strain and Sieber's theory of role accumulation (Lengacher, 1997). The WRSI is a 44-item self-report instrument scored on a 5-point Likert-type scale of "strongly agree" to "strongly disagree." The items are summed to calculate a total women's role strain score, with the higher scores indicating higher role strain experienced by the person (Lengacher, 1997). Cronbach's alpha on the total scale was 0.93 (Lengacher, 1997). The Cronbach alpha for the pilot study and the current study were 0.84 and 0.94 respectively. This scale was found to have good content and construct validity (Lengacher, 1997).

Interpersonal conflict was measured by the Conflict Scale of the Interpersonal Relationships Inventory (IRI; Tilden, Nelson, & Max, 1990). It consists of 13 items scored on a 5-point Likert-type scale rated from "strongly agree" to "strongly disagree." The items are summed to calculate a total conflict score, with increasing scores indicating higher conflict. The internal consistency for the Conflict Scale ranged from 0.81 to 0.91. Two-week test-retest reliability of the Conflict Scale was 0.81. The Conflict Scale was translated into Thai language for use with Thai women. Cronbach's alpha for a pilot study and the current study were 0.84 and 0.92 respectively. This scale was found to have good construct validity (Tilden et al., 1990).

Parental role strain was measured by the Parental Stress Scale (PS). The Parental Stress Scale (PS), developed by Berry and Jones (1995), was designed to assess the level of stress of a person as being a parent. The PS consists of 18 items on a 5-point Likert-type scale rated from "strongly agree" to "strongly disagree." The items are summed to calculate a total parental stress score, with increasing scores indicating higher parental role strain. The internal consistency for the total scale of the PS was 0.83 and item-total correlations ranged from 0.27 to 0.59 (Berry & Jones, 1995). Before being used in the study, the PS was translated into Thai. The Cronbach alpha for the pilot study and the current study were 0.77 and 0.91 respectively. This scale was found to have good construct and criterion validity (Berry & Jones, 1995).

Social support was measured by The Personal Resource Questionnaire (PRQ) Part I & II, developed by Brandt and Weinert in 1981. The PRQ Part I provides descriptive information about the person's resources and their satisfaction with the help they received from their resources (Weinert & Brandt, 1987). Part I consists of 10 life situations in which one might be expected to need some help and information. The social support index for Part I is created by summing the total number of resources the respondent can count on across the 10 life situations. The PRQ Part

II was used to measure a respondent's perceived level of social support consisting of a 25-item, 7-point Likert-type scale rated from "strongly agree" (7) to "strongly disagree" (1). The items were summed to create a total score ranging from 25 to 175 in which higher scores indicate higher levels of perceived social support (Weinert, 1988). PRQ Part I had never been translated into Thai; therefore, it was translated into Thai before being used in the study. PRQ Part II was already translated into Thai and used in some studies in Thailand. After pilot testing, PRQ Part I and II were found to have good reliability and were suitable for use in the study.

Sense of belonging was measured with the Sense of Belonging Instrument, Psychological (SOBI-P; Hagerty & Patusky, 1995). It is designed to measure a person's sense of being valued and their sense of fit within an interpersonal relationship. The SOBI-P is an 18-item, self-report instrument scored on a 4-point Likert-type scale of "strongly agree" to "strongly disagree." The items were summed to calculate a total sense of belonging score, with increasing scores indicating higher sense of belonging. Cronbach's coefficients alpha for the SOBI-P ranges from .91 to .93 demonstrating excellent reliability (Hagerty & Patusky, 1995). The SOBI-P was translated into Thai prior to use in the study. The Cronbach alpha for a pilot study and the current study were 0.89 and 0.98 respectively. This scale was found to have good construct validity (Hagerty & Patusky, 1995).

RESULTS

Data were analyzed using SPSS 9.0 for Windows. Descriptive statistics (e.g., mean, standard deviations, ranges) were used to describe the demographic characteristics of the sample and the major variables of the study. In addition, Pearson correlation coefficients were used to examine the correlations among the variables of the study. Chi-square and logistic regression were used to address hypothesis 1. Logistic regression and *t* tests were used to address hypotheses 2 and 3. For hypotheses 4 to 9, path analysis was used to answer questions regarding the effect of predisposing factors, stressors, and psychosocial factors on severity of depression.

To test for mediation, a series of regression equations were performed: "(a) the outcome variable is regressed on the predictor variable; (b) the mediator is regressed on the predictor variable; and (c) the outcome variable is regressed on the predictor and mediator variables simultaneously" (Lindley & Walker, 1993, p. 278). Separate coefficients for each equation must be estimated and tested (Lindley & Walker, 1993). The mediator function can be confirmed by four conditions:

1. The predictor variable has significant effect on the outcome variable in the first equation;
2. The predictor variable has significant effect on the mediator variable in the second equation;
3. From the equation three, the mediator has significant effect on the outcome variable; and

4. According to equation one and three, the previously significant relationship between the predictor variable and the outcome variable in equation one becomes nonsignificant in equation three (Baron & Kenny, 1986; Lindley & Walker, 1993).

Because path analysis consists of a series of multiple regressions, a multicollinearity diagnostic procedure and scatter plots of residuals were done to confirm that the assumptions of multicollinearity, linearity, normality, and homogeneity of variance for multiple regression were met (Munro, 1997). The results showed that all assumptions except for the assumption for normality were met. Depressive symptom data were not normally distributed and, therefore, transformed using the square root method. After being transformed, the depressive symptom data appeared to be normally distributed.

Hypothesis 1. The results from chi-square analyses showed that depressed women were significantly more likely to have family history of depression (χ^2 = 15.42, $p < .001$) and past history of loss of mother before age 11 ($\chi^2 = 6.53$, $p < .01$) than nondepressed women. Sixteen depressed women had family history of depression and none of the nondepressed women had family history of depression. In addition, results from likelihood-ratio statistics revealed that family history of depression ($\chi^2 = 20.78$, $p < .001$) and past history of loss of mother before age 11 (χ^2 = 6.12, $p < .05$) contributed significantly to prediction of development of depression in Thai women. Therefore, hypothesis 1 was supported.

Hypothesis 2. Results from *t* tests revealed that depressed women scored significantly higher on number of stressful life events ($t = 3.88$, $p < .001$), parental role strain ($t = 2.30$, $p < .05$), interpersonal conflict ($t = 4.79$, $p < .001$), and perceived stress ($t = 6.57$, $p < .001$) than did nondepressed women. However, there was no significant difference on scores of women's role strain ($t = 1.32$, $p = .19$) between depressed and nondepressed women. Therefore, this hypothesis was partially supported. When the path model was examined by logistical regression, results showed that among stress measures, only perceived stress contributed significantly to the prediction of the development of depression in Thai women (Wald statistic = 11.28, $p < .001$).

Hypothesis 3. Results from *t* tests showed that depressed women scored significantly lower on interpersonal resources ($t = 2.19$, $p < .05$), perceived social support ($t = 5.41$, $p < .001$), and sense of belonging ($t = 6.15$, $p < .001$) than did nondepressed women. Therefore, this hypothesis was supported. When the predictor role of these psychosocial factors was examined, results from logistic regression showed that among psychosocial factors, only sense of belonging contributed significantly to the prediction of depression in Thai women (Wald statistic = 8.71, $p = .003$).

Hypotheses 4, 5, 6. The effect of predisposing factors, stressors, and psychosocial factors on severity of depression was examined with path analysis. Results showed that only two variables were found to have direct effect on severity of depression, family history of depression ($\beta = .14$, $p < .05$) and perceived stress ($\beta = .73$, $p <$ $.001$). Therefore, hypotheses 4 and 5 were partially supported and hypothesis 6 was not supported. Results from the path analysis are presented in Table 9.1 and the path model with significant standardized path coefficients is illustrated in Figure 9.2.

Hypotheses 7, 8, 9. These hypotheses related to examining mediation effects. Hypothesis 7: Examining the mediating effect of stressors on predisposing factors and severity of depression, results showed that only perceived stress was found to partially mediate the effect of family history of depression on severity of depression. At step 1, family history of depression had a significant effect on severity of depression ($\beta = .27, p < .05$). At step 2, family history of depression had a significant effect on perceived stress ($\beta = .18, p < .05$). At step 3, when regressing severity of depression on both all predisposing factors and all stressor variables, perceived stress had a significant effect on severity of depression ($\beta = .78, p < .001$) and the effect of family history of depression on severity of depression was reduced from .27 to .14 ($\beta = .27, p < .001$ to $\beta = .14, p < .05$). The hypothesis was partially supported.

Hypothesis 8. The findings portrayed the mediating effect of psychosocial factors on predisposing factors and severity of depression. Results showed that sense of belonging partially mediated the effect of family history of depression on severity of depression. At step 1, family history of depression had a significant effect on severity of depression ($\beta = .27, p < .05$). At step 2, family history of depression had a significant effect on sense of belonging ($\beta = -.19, p < .05$). At step 3, when regressing severity of

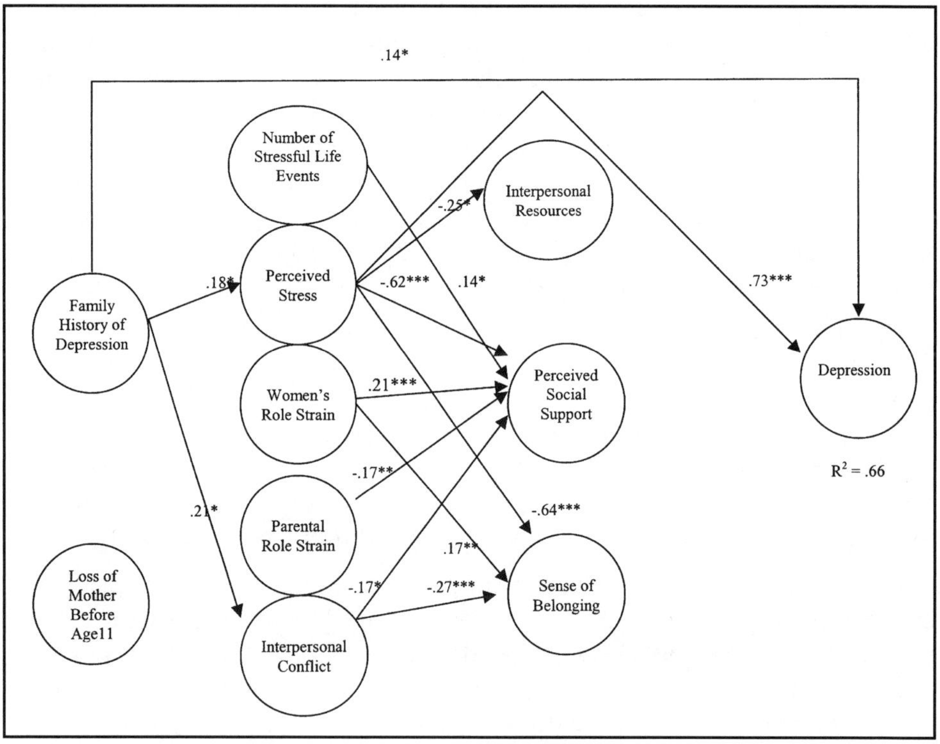

Figure 9.2. Path model with significant standardized path coefficients.

TABLE 9.1. Regression Equations and Path Coefficients

	Equation 1	Equation 2	Equation 3	Equation 4	Equation 5	Equation 6	Equation 7	Equation 8	Equation 9
	Number of Stressful Life Events	Perceived Stress	Interpersonal Conflict	Women's Role Strain	Parental Role Strain	Interpersonal Resources	Perceived Social Support	Sense of Belonging	Depressive Symptoms
Family history of depression	.14	.18*	.21*	.06	.02	.06	-.05	-.03	.14*
Loss of mother before age 11	.06	.07	.11	-.02	.06	-.10	.02	.02	.06
Number of stressful life events						-.04	.14*	.01	.07
Perceived stress						-.25*	-.62***	-.64***	.73***
Interpersonal conflict						.03	-.17*	-.27***	-.11
Women's role strain						.07	.22***	.17**	.01
Parental role strain						-.01	-.17**	.01	-.01
Interpersonal resources									-.01
Perceived social support									-.03
Sense of belonging									-.05
R^2	.02	.04	.06*	.002	.004	.08	.55***	.67***	.66***

Note. Numbers are standardized regression coefficients.
$^*p < .05$. $^{**}p < .01$. $^{***}p < .001$.

depression on both all predisposing factors and all psychosocial variables, sense of belonging had a significant effect on severity of depression ($\beta = -.45, p < .001$) and the effect of family history of depression on severity of depression was reduced from .27 to .15 ($\beta = .27, p < .001$ to $\beta = .15, p < .05$). Thus, this hypothesis was partially supported.

Hypothesis 9. This hypothesis examined the mediating effect of psychosocial factors on stressors and severity of depression. Results revealed that none of the psychosocial factors mediate the effect of stressors on severity of depression. Results from all three steps of multiple regression procedures revealed nonsignificant betas. Thus, this hypothesis was not supported.

DISCUSSION

THE EFFECTS OF PREDISPOSING FACTORS

Family History of Depression. Results indicated that family history of depression was a significant predictor for both having depression and the severity of depression in Thai women. Results from this study in Thailand support the findings in western countries that a family history of depression is an important predictor of depression. Another interesting issue worth noting is the participants' reports about their family histories of depression. Persons who reported that they had a family member with depression were more depressed than persons who reported no family member suffering from depression. It may be that women who suffered or had negative experiences with a depressed family member tended to recall depressed family history and negative experiences more than nondepressed persons with a positive family history. Women who did not have negative experiences with their depressed family member may not have recalled the family member as being depressed.

Loss of Mother Before Age 11. There were differences in results regarding the effects of loss of mother before age 11 on depression in Thai women. When comparing the groups of depressed and nondepressed women, loss of mother before age 11 was a significant predictor of the depressed group. Results from correlations and path analyses, however, failed to support the effect of loss of mother before age 11 on the severity of depression. The results indicated that loss of mother before age 11 did not influence the severity of depression in Thai women. One reason for these findings may be that the loss of mother before age 11 is significant when examined only in comparison to other variables. One potential reason for the findings may be differences in how the child lost the mother, that is, death or type of death, separation by divorce, and abandonment. Thus, for Thai women, it could be useful to examine the reasons for separation because they may have an impact on the psychological well-being of the women.

THE EFFECTS OF STRESSORS

According to the results of this study, depressed women scored significantly higher on number of stressful life events, perceived stress, parental role strain, and interpersonal conflict than did nondepressed women. Yet perceived stress was the only stressor variable in the model that significantly predicted clinical depression in Thai women. In addition, according to results from path analysis and mediating effect analysis, among the stressor variables in the model, only perceived stress had direct effects on severity of depression. Moreover, only perceived stress was found to partially mediate the effect of family history of depression on severity of depression. These findings indicated that perceived stress was a key predictor of clinical depression in Thai women, with increased perceived stress leading to the development of clinical depression. As noted previously, persons with high perceived stress were prone to be clinically depressed. Perceived stress also had the greatest direct effect on severity of depression, both significantly and positively. These findings imply that perceived stress might be an epiphenomenon of depression. Since perceived stress appeared to explain most of the variance in severity of depression, to better understand the effect of other stressor variables, the model should be examined without the influence of stress.

The Effects of Psychosocial Factors

As expected, depressed women scored significantly lower on interpersonal resources, perceived social support and sense of belonging than did nondepressed women. However, among these interpersonal variables, only sense of belonging significantly predicted clinical depression in Thai women in the regression model. When examining for direct effects, none of the interpersonal variables in the model had direct effects on severity of depression. As a mediator, only sense of belonging partially mediated the effect of family history of depression on severity of depression.

Findings indicated that depressed women were more likely to view themselves as having less interpersonal resources, perceived social support, and sense of belonging than nondepressed women. Yet the effects of both interpersonal resources and perceived social support were not strong enough to exert a predictor role on depression in Thai women. Sense of belonging was found to be the only psychosocial factor that contributed significantly to the prediction of depression in Thai women from the logistic regression model. These findings indicate that low sense of belonging can increase the risk of becoming depressed, which makes sense of belonging as too much a significant concept that should be seriously considered when intervening with women experiencing depression.

According to the findings from path analysis, the same suggestion can be applied to explain the failure of psychological factors to exert their effects on severity of depression. As perceived stress appeared to explain most of the variance on severity of depression in the path model, the model should be examined without perceived stress. As a variable, this would remove the strong correlation of perceived stress and depression.

Limitations, Recommendations, Conclusions

There are some limitations in this study. First, this study used a convenience sample, thus limiting generalizability of the results to Thai women living in rural areas of Thailand. Second, insufficient data regarding women's role strain and parental role strain suggested that interpretation of these findings should be considered tentative and future investigation needs to be completed. Third, this study was cross-sectional. Although the cross-sectional design was appropriate for this study, it did not allow interpretation of the findings further than the associations between the variables measured, such as stress and depression. Therefore, a longitudinal design could be useful for future research so that more implications regarding the causal relationship between variables can be examined.

When removing the perceived stress variable in the model, it is possible to exhibit findings that may be more accurate. Replication of the study with a sample of women living in another part of Thailand will increase the generalizability of the results. A longitudinal design could be used to begin investigating the causal relationships between variables in the model.

Findings from this study have important implications for nursing and, in general, health care in Thailand. These findings can be used to enhance knowledge regarding predictors of depression in Thai women, thus illuminating this illness and its predictors. More awareness and recognition of depression in families of depressed women may provide awareness for better assessment, prevention, and intervention for the incapacitating illness.

The findings speak to the importance of information regarding childhood parental loss. In Thailand, little attention has been given to the problem of childhood parental loss and adequate attention should be given to this variable as part of the health assessment.

The findings indicate that the level of perceived stress has a very high correlation with depression in Thai women. This suggests that interventions for women with depression should focus on management of stress as well as alleviation of depression symptoms. Additionally, findings revealed the important role of sense of belonging, suggesting that adequate attention should be given to improving depressed women's sense of belonging.

REFERENCES

Abramis, D. J. (1985). *Job stressors, strains, job performance, social support, and social conflict: Causal relationships in a four-wave longitudinal panel study.* Unpublished doctoral dissertation, University of Michigan, Ann Arbor.

Aneshensel, C. S., & Frerichs, R. R. (1982). Stress, support, and depression: A longitudinal causal model. *Journal of Community Psychology, 10,* 363-376.

Aneshensel, C. S., Frerichs, R. R., & Clark, V. A. (1981). Family roles and sex differences in depression. *Journal of Health and Social Behavior, 22,* 379-393.

Baron, R. M., & Kenny, D. (1986). The moderator-mediator variable distinction in social psychological research: Conceptual, strategies, and statistical considerations. *Journal of Personality and Social Psychology, 51*(6), 1173-1182.

Beeber, L. S. (1987). *The relationship of self-esteem, social support, and depressive symptoms in women.* Unpublished doctoral dissertation, University of Rochester, New York.

Berry, J. O., & Jones, W. H. (1995). The parental stress scale: Initial psychometric evidence. *Journal of Social and Personal Relationships, 12*(3), 463-472.

Blazer, D. G., Kessler, R. C., McGonagle, K. A., & Swartz, M. S. (1994). The prevalence and distribution of major depression in a national community sample: The national comorbidity survey. *American Journal of Psychiatry, 151*(7), 979-986.

Boyce, P., Harris, M., Silove, D., Morgan, N., Wilhelm, A., & Hadzi-Pavlovic, D. (1998). Psychosocial factors associated with depression: A study of socially disadvantaged women with young children. *The Journal of Nervous and Mental Disease, 186*(1), 3-11.

Brown, G. W., Bifulco, A., & Harris, T. O. (1987). Life events, vulnerability, and onset of depression: Some refinements. *British Journal of Psychiatry, 150*, 30-42.

Brown, G. W., & Harris, T. (1978). *Social origins of depression: A study of psychiatric disorder in women.* New York: The Free Press.

Brugha, T. S., Bebbington, P. E., Stretch, D. D., MacCarthy, B., & Wykes, T. (1997). Predicting the short-term outcome of first episodes and recurrences of clinical depression: A prospective study of life events, difficulties, and social support networks. *Journal of Clinical Psychiatry, 58*(7), 298-306.

Brugha, T., Bebbington, P., Tennant, C., & Hurry, J. (1985). The list of threatening experiences: A subset of 12 life events categories with considerable long-term contextual threat. *Psychological Medicine, 15*(1), 189-194.

Cleary, P. D., & Mechanic, D. (1983). Sex differences in psychological distress among married people. *Journal of Health and Social Behavior, 24*, 111-121.

Cohen, J. (1988). *Statistical power analysis for the behavioral sciences.* Hillsdale, NJ: Lawrence Erlbaum.

Cohen, S., Kamarck, T., & Mermelstein, R. (1983). A global measure of perceived stress. *Journal of Health and Social Behavior, 24*, 385-396.

Coyne, J. C., Burchill, S. A., & Stiles, W. B. (1991). An interactional perspective on depression. In C. R. Snyder & D. R. Forsyth (Eds.), *Handbook of social and clinical psychology: The health perspective* (pp. 349-372). New York: Pergamon Press..

Coyne, J. C., & Downey, G. (1991). Social factors and psychopathology: Stress, social support, and coping processes. *Annual Review of Psychology, 42*, 401-425.

Hagerty, B. M., Lynch-Sauer, J., Patusky, K. L., Bouwsema, M., & Collier, P. (1992). Sense of belonging: A vital mental health concept. *Archives of Psychiatric Nursing, 6*(3), 172-177.

Hagerty, B. M., & Patusky, K. (1995). Developing a measure of sense of belonging. *Nursing Research, 44*(1), 9-13.

Hagerty, B. M. K., & Williams, R. A. (1999). The effects of sense of belonging, social support, conflict and loneliness on depression. *Nursing Research, 48*(4), 215-219.

Hagerty, M. B., Williams, R. A., Coyne, J. C., & Early, M. (1996). Sense of belonging and indicators of social and psychological functioning. *Archives of Psychiatric Nursing, 10*(4), 235-244.

Horwath, E., Johmson, J., Klerman, G. L., & Weissman, M. M. (1994). What are the public health implications of subclinical depression symptoms? *Psychiatric Quarterly, 65*(4), 323-337.

Hulin, C. L., Drasgow, F., & Parsons, C. K. (1983). *Item response theory: Application to psychological measurement.* Illinois: Dow Jones-Irwin.

Kendler, K. S., Karkowski, L. M., & Prescott, C. A. (1999). Causal relationship between stressful life events and onset of major depression. *The American Journal of Psychiatry, 156*(6), 837-841.

Kendler, K. S., Kessler, R. C., Neale, M. C., Health, A. C., & Eaves, L. J. (1993). The prediction of major depression in women: Toward an integrated etiologic model. *American Journal of Psychiatry, 150*(8), 1139-1148.

Lengacher, C. A. (1997). A reliablity and validity study of the Women's Role Strain Inventory. *Journal of Nursing Measurement, 5*(2), 139-150.

Lennon, M. C., & Rosenfield, S. (1992). Women and mental health: The interaction of job and family conditions. *Journal of Health and Social Behavior, 33*, 316-327.

Lewinsohn, P. M., & Hoberman, H. M. (1988). A prospective study of risk factors for unipolar depression. *Journal of Abnormal Psychology, 97*(3), 251-264.

Lindley, P., & Walker, S. N. (1993). Theoretical and methodological differentiation of moderation and mediation. *Nursing Research, 42*(5), 276-279.

Lotrakul, M., & Sukanich, P. (1999). Development of the Thai Depression Inventory. *Journal of Medical Association of Thailand, 82*, 1200-1207.

McGrath, E., Keita, G. P., Strickland, B. R., & Russo, N. F. (1990). *Women and depression: Risk factors and treatment issues.* Washington, DC: American Psychological Association.

Mental Health Department. (1997). *Mental health development plan: Follow the eighth national social and economic development plan, 1997-2001.* Nonthaburi, Thailand: Author.

Monroe, S. M., Connell, M. M., Bromet, E. J., & Steiner, S. C. (1986). Social support, life events, and depressive symptoms: A 1-year prospective study. *Journal of Consulting and Clinical Psychology, 54*(4), 424-431.

Munro, B. H. (1997). Regression. In B. H. Munro (Ed.), *Statistical methods for health care research* (3rd ed.). New York: Lippincott.

Murray, C. J. L., & Lopaz, A. D. (1996). Alternative visions of the future: Projecting mortality and disability, 1990-2020. In C. J. L. Murray & A. D. Lopez (Eds.), *The global burden of disease* (pp. 325-395). Boston, MA: The Harvard School of Public Health on the behalf of The World Health Organization and The World Bank.

Nolen-Hoeksema, S. (1987). Sex differences in unipolar depression: Evidence and theory. *Psychological Bulletin, 101,* 259-282.

Nolen-Hoeksema, S. (1990). *Sex differences in depression.* California: Stanford University Press.

Nolen-Hoeksema, S. (1995). Epidemiology and theories of gender differences in unipolar depression. In S. M. Violette (Ed.), *Gender and psychopathology* (pp. 63-87). Washington, DC: American Psychiatric Press.

Paykel, E. S. (1994). Life events, social support and depression. *Acta Psychiatrica Scandinavica, 377* (Suppl.), 50-58.

Spielmann, S. (1994). The family in Thailand and drug demand reduction: Problems of urban Thai society in transaction. *Bulletin on Narcotics, 46*(1), 45-66.

Stuart, G. W. (1981). Role strain and depression: A causal inquiry. *Journal of Psychosocial Nursing and Mental Health Services, 19*(12), 20-28.

Stuart, G. W. (1995). Emotional responses and mood disorders. In G. W. Stuart & S. J. Sundeen (Eds.), *Principles & practice of psychiatric nursing* (5th ed., pp. 1021). Baltimore: Mosby.

Tiedje, L. B. C. (1987). *Multiple role women: Inter-role compatibility perceptions and coping effectiveness and adjustment.* Unpublished doctoral dissertation, University of Michigan, Ann Arbor.

Tilden, V. P., Nelson, C. A., & May, B. A. (1990). The IPR Inventory: Development and psychometric characteristics. *Nursing Research, 39*(6), 337-343.

Warren, B. J. (1995). *Constructing a model for depression in middle class African-American women by exploring relationships between life events, social support, and self-esteem.* Unpublished doctoral dissertation, The Ohio State University, Columbus.

Weinert, C. (1988). Measuring social support: Revision and future development of the personal resource questionnaire. In C. F. Waltz & O. L. Strickland (Eds.), *Measurement of nursing outcomes* (Vol. 1, pp. 309-327). New York: Springer Publishing.

Weinert, C., & Brandt, P. A. (1987). Measuring social support with the personal resource questionnaire. *Western Journal of Nursing Research, 9*(4), 589-602.

Weissman, M. M., & Olfson, M. (1995). Depression in women: Implications for health care research. *Science, 269,* 799-801.

Yoddumnern-Attig, B., Richer, K., Soonthorndhada, A., Sethaput, C., & Pramualratana, A. (1992). *Changing roles and statuses of women in Thailand: A documentary assessment.* Nakhonpathom, Thailand: The Institute for Population and Social Research, Mahidol University at Salaya.

Zauszniewski, J. A. (1994). Potential sequelae of family history of depression: Identifying family members at risk. *Journal of Psychosocial Nursing and Mental Health Services, 32*(9), 15-21.

10

Depression Coping Self-Efficacy as a Predictor of Relapse 1 and 2 Years Following Psychiatric Hospital-Based Treatment

Sharon Tucker
Susan Brust
Pamela Pierce
Carol Fristedt
V. Shane Pankratz

Depression is a serious and disabling illness for many people resulting in enormous suffering, poor quality of life, lost productivity, family conflict and suffering, and in some cases suicide. Numerous effective treatment options and settings are available including psychopharmacologic and other biologic and somatic and psychological treatments delivered through a variety of modalities. The limited longitudinal studies available indicate that despite these multiple treatment options, relapse in the initial 2 years following treatment is common. The evidence indicates that about 25% to 40% of individuals who are treated for a first episode of depression relapse in this time interval (Keller & Boland, 1998; Lin et al., 1998; Quiring, Monroe, Simons, & Thase, 2002; Simon et al., 2002). Moreover, for each subsequent episode of depression, the interval between episodes has been shown to decrease (Keller & Boland, 1998). One study suggests that, for those with a history of recurrent depression, the risk for relapse during 2 years of follow-up exceeds 75% (Frank et al., 1990). Unsuccessful treatment of depression and/or multiple relapses are markers of chronic depression, which affects approximately 10% of persons who experience depression (Lin et al., 1998).

Numerous factors have been associated with relapse. They include history of multiple episodes, double depression (dysthymia and major depression), onset after age 60, long duration of individual episodes, family history of affective disorder, comorbid anxiety disorder or substance abuse, and poor symptom control during continuation therapy (Keller & Boland, 1998). A dimension of symptom control that has not been well studied with the depressed population, but may prove to be a predictor of relapse, is depression coping self-efficacy. Depression coping self-efficacy builds on Bandura's theory of self-efficacy (Bandura, 1977) and represents one's perception or judgment about one's ability to manage depressive symptoms and the treatments recommended for recovery (Perraud, 2000). Although depression coping self-efficacy has received very little study, self-efficacy related to other health conditions such as weight control, smoking cessation, pain control, and coronary heart disease has been examined (Bandura, 1997; Bernier & Avard, 1986; Condiotte & Lichtenstein, 1981; Dolce, 1987; Sullivan, LaCroix, Russo, & Katon, 1998). Findings have suggested that higher self-efficacy predicts better performance. However, a limitation to a majority of these studies is the fact that the follow-up periods have been short, typically only 3 to 6 months. The study of depression coping self-efficacy related to dealing with the effects of depression and its management is a novel direction that may help guide the treatment of depression as well as predict who is at greatest risk for relapse. This study examined depression coping self-efficacy and its relationship with recovery and relapse over a 2-year period following an index depressive episode and the subsequent hospital-based treatment of the episode.

PURPOSE

The primary purposes of this longitudinal study were to: (a) compare depressive symptom and depression coping self-efficacy scores at 2-years posttreatment with scores reported at completion of treatment and (b) examine posttreatment depression coping self-efficacy scores as a predictor of greater frequencies of health care visits, including rehospitalization, during a period of 2 years following treatment, among participants treated for depression in a hospital-based treatment program. The study that provided the participants for this longitudinal follow-up had evaluated 2 treatment modalities, with an equal number of patients originally treated either as inpatients or in a partial hospital program (PHP). Therefore, a secondary purpose was to examine if depression coping self-efficacy and depressive symptoms in study participants differed at 2 years as a function of type of original treatment.

METHOD

DESIGN

A longitudinal design with two components was used to examine the research aims. Both components were descriptive and correlational in nature. The first comprised a year of passive follow-up through a retrospective review of the medical records of participants treated for depression. Frequencies and types of health care visits sought by participants over the 1 year since treatment were abstracted from the health care records. The second component consisted of a 2-year follow-up, in which the same participants were contacted at their homes through the mail and invited to complete and return a collection of three surveys. These surveys asked questions regarding participant depression coping self-efficacy, depressive symptoms, and use of health care services since their index treatment experience of 2 years earlier.

Sample and Setting

The study included a convenience sample of patients with a depressive disorder who were treated at a psychiatric inpatient or PHP at a large midwestern medical center that provided several levels of psychiatric treatment. The inpatient treatment program was a 22-bed unit that is designed to provide crisis intervention for acutely ill psychiatric patients. This program focused on stabilizing symptoms, managing crisis situations, providing mental and physical health education, and arranging less intensive services. The PHP program included two program levels (see Tucker, Brust, & Richardson, 2002) and provided a wide range of services with the overall goal of diverting inpatient treatment to alternative services whenever possible. The inpatient and partial programs offered structured treatment including daily mental health education, supportive group therapy, 1:1 crisis support, family counseling and intervention, milieu therapy, medication therapy, and occupational therapy. The original design recruited a total of 50 participants, with equal numbers being enrolled in each of the two treatment modalities: inpatient or PHP. As the original study was an evaluation design and not a controlled randomized trial, completion of treatment was based on clinician assessment and judgment. Treatment duration was therefore variable among participants.

Inclusion criteria included participants who were at least 18 years old, spoke English, were able to give informed consent, had no history of documented developmental disability and had received at least 48 hours of treatment for a primary diagnosis of a Major Depressive Disorder, Adjustment Disorder with Depressed Mood, or Dysthymic Disorder. Participants were excluded if they had a documented developmental disability, were psychotic, or received less than 48 hours of treatment.

For the 1-year follow-up, 49 of the 50 potential participants (98%) had provided authorization that allowed the retrospective review of their medical records for research purposes. For the 2-year follow-up, all 50 participants were invited through a mailed survey packet to participate, with 26 (52%) participants returning the completed surveys.

Variables and Instruments

The variables of interest in this follow-up study were depression coping self-efficacy, depressive symptoms, and health care visit types and frequencies. Each of these variables and associated instruments is described below.

Depression Coping Self-Efficacy. Depression coping self-efficacy is defined as a person's confidence in their ability to perform tasks designed to provide some control over depressive symptoms (Perraud, 2000). Perraud developed and tested the

Depression Coping Self-Efficacy Scale (DCSES) to measure patients' self-efficacy in their ability to manage and treat their depressive symptoms. The DCSES is a 24-item summated rating scale with response format on a continuum of 0 to 100 (higher scores reflecting more self-efficacy or confidence). Patients are asked to rate their degree of confidence or self-efficacy in managing tasks specific to coping with symptoms of and treatment for depression. Perraud originally tested the DCSES among 150 depressed inpatients and 24 nondepressed community volunteers (Perraud, 2000). DCSES scores were correlated with depression levels as measured by the Beck Depression Inventory and discriminated depressed from nondepressed participants. Tucker and colleagues (2002) further tested the DCSES by examining construct validity of the DCSES among 25 participants receiving inpatient treatment and 25 participants seeking PHP treatment for a depressive disorder. Measures used in their study included both self-report and clinician-rated measures. Findings indicated the DCSES was correlated with levels of depressive symptoms and global functioning. In both studies, internal consistency was demonstrated (Cronbach's alpha coefficients ranged from .91 to .97). Cronbach's alpha coefficient in the current follow-up study was .95.

Depressive Symptoms. Depressive symptoms, reflected in mood, behavior, cognition, and social interactions, were measured using the Center For Epidemiologic Studies Depression (CES-D) Scale (Devons et al., 1988). The CES-D Scale is a 20-item self-report measure of depressive symptomatology intended for use in the general population. Participants rate the extent to which they have experienced symptoms (related to depressed mood, feelings of guilt, worthlessness, loneliness, hopelessness, psychomotor retardation, and disturbances in sleep, concentration, and appetite) over the past week. Summed scores range from 0 to 60. A score of 16 or greater is indicative of depression. Reliability and validity estimates as a screening instrument have been demonstrated (Devons et al., 1988). Cronbach's alpha coefficients for the two treatment groups at baseline and posttreatment ranged from .90 to .95.

Types and Frequencies of Health Care Visits. A major variable of interest was the types and frequencies of health care visits sought by participants following treatment of their index episode. For the 1 year follow-up, health care visits were abstracted from the medical record from one institution and coded as representing encounters and episodes and as psychiatric or nonpsychiatric visits. Health care visits that represented extended treatment experiences such as a hospital stay or PHP treatment or where the treatment was given over a period of days or visits such as a course of outpatient ECT or physical therapy were recorded as health care episodes. Health care visits that were outpatient in nature and appeared to be one-time visits or several discrete visits in which the focus of the multiple visits could not be conclusively determined to be specifically related to a single episode of care were recorded as health care encounters.

The Healthcare Visits Data Recording Form (HVDRF) was designed and used by the researchers to record types and frequencies of health care visits (encounters and episodes) abstracted from medical records of the study institution. The following health care visits data were abstracted from participant medical records:

date(s) for the health care visits, type of health care visits, and presenting problem(s). To ensure rater reliability in abstracting health care visit data from the medical records, two study investigators each reviewed five records individually with pertinent study participant data abstracted and recorded on the HVDRF. Interrater agreement on participant data abstracted from medical records was then evaluated on the five records. Continued training occurred until the raters reached a 90% agreement rate on two consecutive records.

For the 2-year follow-up, the study researchers designed a Two-Year Follow-Up Questionnaire to collect information from participants on the treatments they had received following their treatment of 2 years prior. Participants were asked to report all rehospitalizations for psychiatric or medical problems, the dates of each rehospitalization, and the length of each hospital stay; and all other psychiatric treatments sought over the 2-year period including individual therapy, couples and group psychotherapy, day hospital or partial hospital treatments, and outpatient electroconvulsive therapy (ECT). Content validity was addressed through expert feedback from three doctorally prepared nurses, two of whom specialized in psychiatric nursing.

Procedures

Approval to conduct the study was obtained from the Nursing Research Committee and Institutional Review Board (IRB) of the participating institution. For the 1-year follow-up, the researchers reviewed the medical records of the 49 participants who had authorized use of their medical records for research. All health care visits sought by the participants over the 1 year since treatment were abstracted onto the HVDRF. Baseline and posttreatment scores for the DCSES, CES-D scale, and other demographic and clinical data (age, gender, psychiatric diagnoses, and researcher-rated functioning and symptom distress scores) were abstracted from the original treatment study database and exported into the follow-up study database.

Data recorded on the HVDRF were first coded into type of specialty visits: gynecology, gastrointestinal, preventive medicine, physical medicine and rehabilitation, family medicine, urgent care/emergency room, community internal medicine, inpatient psychiatry, partial psychiatric hospital, group therapy, individual therapy, electroconvulsive therapy, and other. As defined earlier, within each of these specialty categories, the type of visit was categorized as an "encounter" or "episode."

For the 2-year follow-up, 50 participants were invited through the mail to participate in a study to examine their depressive symptoms and coping 2 years following treatment. Survey packets included three surveys (DCSES, CES-D Scale, and Two-Year Follow-Up Questionnaire) and a cover letter explaining the purpose of the follow-up study and participants' right to decline participation without penalty. Participants who had not returned the completed surveys within 2 weeks after the first mailing were sent a second packet. A final reminder letter was sent 2 weeks after the second mailing to those participants who had not yet returned the surveys.

DATA ANALYSIS

Demographic, Depression, and Depression Coping Self-Efficacy Data. Demographic information, including sex, age, alcohol use, and Axis 2 diagnoses, were summarized for those participating in the 1-year and the 2-year follow-up components of the study. Demographic and other baseline summary data, particularly baseline and posttreatment DCSES and CES-D scores, were compared between those who responded to the 2-year follow-up mailings. Comparisons of categorical variables were made using Fisher's exact test. Comparisons between continuous variables were achieved via Mann-Whitney rank sum tests. Depression coping self-efficacy and depressive symptoms at baseline, at posttreatment, and at 2-year follow-up were also summarized. Comparisons between posttreatment DCSES and CES-D Scale scores and their corresponding 2-year follow-up measures were made using Wilcoxon signed rank tests.

Health Care Visits Data. Frequencies and types of health care visits sought by study participants during the two follow-up periods were also summarized. For the 1-year follow-up, all visits noted in the medical record were collated into one of four categories. These categories represented psychiatric versus nonpsychiatric visits, combined with encounters versus episodes, as defined previously. All medical specialty visits were combined into a single group and labeled as nonpsychiatric encounters or episodes. All psychiatric visits were combined and labeled psychiatric encounters or episodes. Frequencies and percentages, and other summary statistics, were then calculated for psychiatric and nonpsychiatric encounters and episodes. For the 2-year follow-up, frequencies and percentages of specific types of outpatient and inpatient visits (psychiatric and nonpsychiatric) were calculated.

Associations Between Depression Coping Self-Efficacy and Health Care Visit Frequencies. The relationships between depression coping self-efficacy scores at time of treatment and the frequencies and types of health care visits sought by study participants over the course of follow-up were examined. Because the frequencies of health care episodes and encounters observed over the first year of follow-up were measured as "count" data, they did not meet assumptions required by standard linear regression methodologies. Therefore, Poisson regression models were used to examine the relationships between frequencies of encounters and episodes and the baseline and posttreatment DCSES scores. Several other variables, demographic and otherwise, were included in the models to examine depression coping self-efficacy as a predictor of subsequent health care visit frequencies after adjusting for other potential correlates of health care visit frequency. These other variables included baseline and posttreatment CES-D scores, baseline and posttreatment researcher-rated participant functioning and symptom distress scores (not a focus in this study; see Tucker et al., 2002, for more detail), psychiatric diagnoses, age, gender, and type of treatment (inpatient or PHP treatment). Exponentiated regression parameters and their 95% confidence intervals (CIs) were computed to summarize the magnitude of the associations between the DCSES, and other variables, and the number of health care episodes or encounters. These estimates reflect the relative frequency of health care episodes or encounters between individuals who differ on an independent variable, such as the DCSES score, by a fixed amount. Spearman rank correlation coefficients were also computed as an additional measure of the strength of the associations between health care episodes or encounters and the independent variables of interest. For the 2-year follow-up data, tests of differences in scores on the DCSES and CES-D Scale were computed between those reporting hospital readmissions and those not reporting readmissions.

Comparisons by Original Study Treatment Group. Data summaries and statistical comparisons were performed separately for the two treatment programs in order to account for the original study design. Potential differences in depression coping self-efficacy and depressive symptom scores at 2 years posttreatment were compared between the two treatment groups. These comparisons were made using Mann-Whitney rank sum tests. All statistical analyses were performed using the SAS software package.

RESULTS

Participant Demographic Summaries

The 49 participants in the 1-year follow-up were 36 (73%) females and 13 (27%) males who ranged in age from 21 to 84 with a mean age of 38.49 (*SD* = 14.12). Psychiatric diagnoses were abstracted from participant medical records. These diagnoses were documented by clinicians at time of treatment using the multiaxial classification system in the *Diagnostic and Statistical Manual of Mental Disorders* (DSM-IV; American Psychiatric Association, 1994). Axis I diagnoses included major depression or a related depressive disorder. A diagnosis of alcohol abuse or dependence was documented on Axis I. Axis II diagnoses included personality problem traits or personality disorders documented by clinicians. Twenty-three (47%) of the total participants were given a diagnosis of a personality trait or disorder: 14 (29%) were identified as having disorders and 9 (18%) as having traits. Thirty-six (73%) of the participants had one or more Axis III diagnoses, that is, medical problems.

Twenty-six (52%) of the 50 participants completed and returned the 2-year follow-up surveys, 2 (4%) participants declined participation, 3 (6%) packets were returned as undeliverable, 1 (2%) survey packet was returned by a family member with a note indicating the participant had committed suicide, and 18 (36%) participants did not respond. The participants who responded ranged in age from 21 to 84 with a mean age of 43.9 (*SD* = 16.2). There were 24 (92.3%) women and 2 (7.7%) men and all 26 were Caucasian.

Table 10.1 contains summaries of the baseline information of study participants, classified according to their participation in the 2-year mailed follow-up. The table includes demographic data (age, gender, treatment group, and diagnosis) and the baseline and posttreatment means and standard deviations for the DCSES and CES-D Scale. As reported in a previous publication (Tucker et al., 2002), DCSES and CES-D scale scores (inpatient, PHP, and combined) increased significantly from baseline

TABLE 10.1. Baseline and Posttreatment Characteristics of Inpatient and PHP Study Participants Categorized by 2-Year Responders and Nonresponders

	Inpatient						
	Responders (n = 11)			Nonresponders (n = 14)			
	n		(%)	n		(%)	p-value[a]
Female	10		(91)	5		(36)	0.011
ETOH use	1		(9)	8		(57)	0.033
Axis 2 diagnoses							
None	4		(36)	7		(50)	0.584
Traits	3		(27)	5		(36)	
Disorders	4		(36)	2		(14)	
	M	±	SD	M	±	SD	p-value[a]
Age	41.5	±	16.4	37.9	±	12.8	0.722
Baseline							
DCSES	35.8	±	15.7	46.3	±	24.2	0.369
CES-D	41.8	±	10.9	41.8	±	14.8	0.701
Posttreatment							
DCSES	55.0	±	19.1	67.3	±	26.1	0.106
CES-D	32.1	±	15.0	25.0	±	16.2	0.217
	PHP						
	Responders (n = 15)			Nonresponders (n = 10)			
	n		(%)	n		(%)	p-value
Female	14		(93)	8		(80)	0.544
ETOH use	1		(7)	1		(10)	1.000
Axis 2 diagnoses[c]							
None	9		(64)	6		(60)	0.191
Traits	2		(14)	4		(40)	
Disorders	3		(21)	0		(0)	
	M	±	SD	M	±	SD	p-value[a]
Age	45.9	±	15.5	41.7	±	10.9	0.803
Baseline							
DCSES	42.4	±	13.3[b]	46.8	±	18.5	0.364
CES-D	37.5	±	8.5	42.1	±	12.2	0.192
Posttreatment							
DCSES	64.4	±	18.7[b]	71.4	±	17.6	0.402
CES-D	18.9	±	13.9[b]	25.3	±	16.0	0.322

Note. Responders are those who participated in the 2-year follow-up.

[a]p values regard tests of differences between 2-year responders and nonresponders.

[b]Not all participants completed all self-report measures at baseline. One of the inpatients who responded at the 2-year follow-up did not complete the baseline DCSES. Of those in the PHP respondent group, 1 did not complete the baseline DCSES, 2 did not complete the posttreatment DCSES, and 3 did not complete the posttreatment CES-D.

[c]Axis 2 diagnoses were not available for 1 participant due to research authorization refusal for research medical record review.

to posttreatment, demonstrating increased depression coping self-efficacy levels and reduced depressive symptoms following treatment.

Health Care Visit Frequencies and Depression Symptoms/Coping Self-Efficacy Summaries

For all participants over the first year of follow-up, the mean number of psychiatric encounters was 11.2 (*SD* = 17.9) and the mean number of nonpsychiatric encounters was 7.9 (*SD* = 10.7). Ten PHP patients (42%) and 7 inpatients (28%) experienced no psychiatric episodes, 8 (33%) PHP and 8 (32%) inpatient participants had one psychiatric episode, 5 (21%) and 7 (28%) had 2 to 3 psychiatric episodes, and 1 (4%) and 3 (12%) had 4 to 8 psychiatric episodes. The vast majority of participants, 21 (88%) of the PHP patients and 23 (92%) of the inpatients, experienced no nonpsychiatric episodes. Table 10.2 presents for each treatment group the means, standard deviations, median, and maximum values of the number of psychiatric and nonpsychiatric episodes and encounters sought by the study participants during the first year following treatment as abstracted from medical records.

Table 10.3 contains summaries of DCSES scores at the 2-year mailed follow-up, along with average differences from posttreatment to follow-up, categorized by treatment group. Mean DCSES scores 2 years after treatment increased slightly from 55.0 at posttreatment to 60.4 at follow-up for inpatients and decreased slightly from 64.4 at posttreatment to 59.4 at follow-up for PHP participants. These differences in scores from posttreatment to follow-up for the DCSES were not statistically significant for either group ($p = 0.513$ for the inpatient group and $p = 0.541$ for the PHP group).

Per report of a family member, the 1 participant who committed suicide was readmitted to another inpatient unit shortly after treatment and committed suicide within 2 months of the index treatment. This participant's posttreatment DCSES score was 57, which was a 16-point deterioration from the baseline score of 73.

Table 10.3 also contains summaries of CES-D scores at the 2-year mailed follow-up, along with average differences from posttreatment to follow-up categorized by treatment group. Mean CES-D Scale scores 2 years after treatment decreased

TABLE 10.2. Healthcare Episodes and Encounters at 1 Year, Abstracted Via Medical Record Review, Categorized by Initial Treatment Group

	Medical Record Review					
	Inpatient (*n* = 25)			PHP (*n* = 24)		
	M ± *SD*	*Mdn*	Max	*M* ± *SD*	*Mdn*	Max
Psychiatric						
Episodes	1.8 ± 2.0	1	8	1.1 ± 1.6	1.0	7
Encounters	4.0 ± 8.4	0	36	18.6 ± 22.0	13.0	91
Non-psychiatric						
Episodes	0.1 ± 0.3	0	1	0.1 ± 0.3	0.0	1
Encounters	3.7 ± 6.0	0	19	12.3 ± 12.7	8.5	43

TABLE 10.3. Two-Year Follow-Up Mean DCSES and CES-D Scores and Change Scores for Each Treatment Group

	Inpatient (n = 11)		
	Follow-up	Change[a]	
	$M \pm SD$	$M \pm SD$	p-value[b]
DCSES	60.4 ± 26.8	5.4 ± 26.2	0.513
CES-D	22.7 ± 20.2	-9.4 ± 19.9	0.149
	PHP (n = 15)		
	Follow-up	Change[a]	
	$M \pm SD$	$M \pm SD$	p-value[b]
DCSES	59.4 ± 14.9	-3.8 ± 22.0	0.541
CES-D	20.9 ± 8.7	1.6 ± 13.6	0.694

[a]p values regard test of change from posttreatment to follow-up.
[b]Follow-up posttreatment.

from 32.1 at posttreatment to 22.7 at follow-up for inpatients and increased from 18.9 at posttreatment to 20.9 at follow-up for PHP participants. These differences did not reach statistical significance (p = 0.149 for the inpatient group and 0.694 for the PHP group).

The 1 participant who committed suicide had reported a degree of depressive symptoms that was of clinical concern at both baseline and posttreatment. This patient's CES-D scale score of 34 both at baseline and posttreatment was markedly higher than the typical cutoff value of 16 on the CES-D scale.

At the 2-year follow-up, participants self-reported both outpatient and inpatient treatments received since their index treatment experience of 2 years earlier. Regarding the 11 inpatient participant responders, 7 (64%) reported they had received individual therapy, 2 (18%) group therapy, 2 (18%) family therapy, 2 (18%) intense outpatient therapy, 1 (9%) PHP or day treatment, and 1 (9%) electroconvulsive therapy. Among the 15 PHP participant responders, 10 (67%) reported they had received individual therapy; 5 (33%) group therapy; 2 (13%) electroconvulsive therapy; and 1 (7%) each for family therapy, intense outpatient therapy, and PHP or day treatment.

The 2-year follow-up participants also identified rehospitalizations for psychiatric and medical problems following their index treatment for depression. Psychiatric rehospitalizations were for depression, anxiety, suicidal thoughts, suicide attempts, and alcohol and drug use. Among the 11 inpatient participant responders, 5 (45%) reported 1 or more inpatient readmissions during the follow-up period, for a total of 21 psychiatric readmissions and 3 readmissions for other medical problems. Among the 15 PHP participant responders, 6 (40%) reported one or more readmissions during the follow-up period, for a total of 13 psychiatric readmissions and 4 readmissions for other medical problems.

Associations Between Depression Coping Self-efficacy and Health Care Visit Frequencies

There were no significant associations between posttreatment DCSES scores with 1-year follow-up encounters of psychiatric and nonpsychiatric care or of nonpsychiatric episodes of care, when using Poisson regression to perform the statistical comparisons. Yet there was a significant Spearman's rank correlation coefficient of -0.34 (95% *CI*: -0.57 to -0.05, p = .021), which suggested a moderate negative association between posttreatment DCSES scores and the number of episodes of psychiatric care during the first year of follow-up.

To further examine the significance of associations between depression coping self-efficacy scores and frequencies of psychiatric episodes, additional variables that might have been associated with greater frequencies of psychiatric episodes over the first follow-up year were also examined in Poisson regression models. The variables in the models included age, gender, group status (inpatient vs. PHP status), Axis I major psychiatric disorder including alcohol use problems, Axis II traits or disorders, baseline and posttreatment DCSES scores, baseline and posttreatment scores from the CES-D scale, and baseline and posttreatment functioning and symptom distress ratings provided by study researchers. None of these variables reached statistical significance in this relatively small sample of 49 participants.

For the 2-year follow-up, participants who reported psychiatric rehospitalizations were compared to those who did not. As outlined in Table 10.4, 8 (31%) of the 26 2-year responders self-reported one or more rehospitalizations for psychiatric illness. The average 2-year follow-up DCSES score among the 18 respondents who did not report psychiatric hospitalizations was 63.7 (*SD* = 19.7) while the average DCSES score of the 8 who did report psychiatric hospitalizations was 51.1 (*SD* = 20.1). The mean 2-year follow-up CES-D scores were 19.8 (*SD* = 13.0) and 25.8 (*SD* = 17.3) for those who did not and those who did report psychiatric rehospitalization, respectively. These differences were not statistically significant (DCSES: p = 0.330, CES-D: p = 0.597).

Among the 8 participants who reported psychiatric rehospitalizations, 6 reported two or more psychiatric rehospitalizations. The mean posttreatment DCSES score for these 6 participants was 50.2 (*SD* = 20.9), compared to the mean posttreatment DCSES score of 60.6 (*SD* = 16.9) for those reporting no rehospitalizations.

Comparisons By Original Study Treatment Group

A secondary purpose of the study was to compare DCSES and CES-D Scale scores between original study treatment groups at 2 years posttreatment. As observed in Table 10.3, the DCSES and CES-D scores were similar between inpatients and those in the PHP group. Comparisons between the two treatment groups at 2 years posttreatment did not reach statistical significance (p = 1.000 for the DCSES and 0.78 for the CES-D scale).

TABLE 10.4. Posttreatment and Follow-Up DCSES Scores for the 8 Individual Participants Who Self-Reported Hospital Readmissions During the 2-Year Follow-Up Period

	DCSES Scores		Number & Type of
Treatment Group	Posttreatment	2-Year Follow-Up	Hospital Readmissions
PHP	65	59	7 psychiatric
PHP	25	68	2 psychiatric & 1 medical
PHP	58	40	3 psychiatric
PHP	83	70	1 psychiatric
Inpatient	88	63	1 psychiatric
Inpatient	30	8	2 psychiatric
Inpatient	44	49	9 psychiatric
Inpatient	79	52	9 psychiatric & 2 medical

DISCUSSION

Depression is a serious illness and leading cause of disability in the United States and worldwide (National Institute of Mental Health, 2000). It is estimated that 5% to 20% of people will suffer from depression at least once in their lives with higher rates among select groups including females and those with comorbidities (Doris, Ebmeier, & Shajahan, 1999; Keller & Boland, 1998; Kessler et al., 1994; Kessler, Zhao, Blazer, & Swartz, 1997; Lin et al., 1998; Quiring et al., 2002; Simon et al., 2002; Weissman et al., 1996). Although effective treatment with complete recovery is achievable for about 80% of those suffering from depression (Keller & Boland, 1998), relapse rates within the first 2 years of an index episode are reported to range from 20% to 40%.

The relapse rate for the participants in this study was very consistent with previous reports particularly for a group with significant comorbidities. At time of treatment, nearly 1/2 the sample was given a diagnosis of a personality disorder or trait (Axis II) and 3/4 were diagnosed with one or more medical conditions (Axis III). The outcomes measured from pretreatment to 2-years posttreatment also point to the chronicity of these participants. Despite 2-year maintenance of significant improvements in depression coping self-efficacy, depressive symptoms, and functioning following treatment, the mean depressive symptom scores reported by participants remained above cutoff scores on the CES-D scale. Moreover, 2/3 of the sample had one or more episodes of psychiatric care over the year following their treatment and over 1/4 of the participants were rehospitalized for psychiatric illness.

In addition to comorbidities, a number of other factors have been found to predict depression relapse and poor response to treatment. Among these factors are multiple episodes, family history of affective disorder, long duration of episodes, and poor symptom control in continuation therapy (Keller & Boland, 1998). A dimension of symptom control, depression coping self-efficacy, was examined in this study as a predictor of greater frequencies of health care visits following treatment. Depression coping self-efficacy is defined as depressed persons' judgment of their ability to manage their symptoms and the strategies recommended to treat the symptoms. Consistent with self-efficacy theory and research on other health conditions where self-efficacy has predicted health behavior change, the investigators postulated that depression coping self-efficacy may predict performance related to symptom management and risk for relapse. Thus, depressed persons with greater depression coping self-efficacy were expected to actively follow their treatment regimen, persist when the recovery process seems stalled, avoid self-denigrating attributions, and experience low to moderate anxiety. The converse was expected for persons with low depression coping self-efficacy, leaving them more vulnerable to relapse and in need of further intense treatment.

The 1-year study findings did lend partial support to this hypothesis, with the univariate association between posttreatment DCSES scores and the number of episodes of care in the year following treatment. However, the Poisson regression models did not reach statistical significance. The difference between these two analytical results may be related to how the numbers of encounters and episodes were defined and measured, which resulted in significant Poisson overdispersion of the recorded numbers of encounters and episodes. The univariate correlations were computed in a nonparametric fashion and were therefore not subject to distributional assumptions. The fact that depression coping self-efficacy scores at posttreatment correlated with psychiatric episodes of care during the year following treatment indicates that further research is warranted. Moreover, the DCSES was the only variable among several to correlate significantly with psychiatric episodes of care over 1 year following treatment. Lower DCSES scores at time of posttreatment from the original treatment program were found among those participants who had more episodes of psychiatric treatment in the first year following treatment. This finding, while moderate and tentative, extends previous research on self-efficacy related to other health conditions. It also offers longitudinal data beyond 6 months, which are missing from most studies examining self-efficacy and health behaviors.

The 2-year self-reported findings indicated posttreatment DCSES scores were not statistically significant different between those who reported repeat hospitalizations for psychiatric care and those who reported no rehospitalizations. However, the statistical power to detect differences was only 29% and the actual score differences were in the expected directions. Thus, depression coping self-efficacy levels, measured by the DCSES, may predict who is at greatest risk of relapse at least within the first year following treatment. Posthospital treatment for such patients may require a different type of posthospital treatment such as continued intensive outpatient assessment or case management with a focus on strengthening depression coping self-efficacy.

A secondary purpose of this study was to examine if 2-year posttreatment depression coping self-efficacy scores differed as a function of original treatment type.

The results from this study did not support inpatient or PHP treatment as preferable for better follow-up outcomes. The groups were fairly comparable in terms of effects on depressive symptoms and increasing depression coping self-efficacy. These findings are consistent with reports from other investigators who have reported similar outcomes (e.g., mental health service contacts, re-hospitalizations, and patient or family ratings of their psychiatric status) for inpatient and partial hospital treatments programs for depression (Kluiter, Giel, Nienhuis, Ruphan, & Wiersma, 1992). Thus, specific targets of treatment may be more important in achieving desired outcomes than actual setting of treatment. Depression coping self-efficacy as a possible target of treatment and predictor of those at greatest risk of relapse warrants further study.

Future research on the DCSES as a predictor of relapse must address the limitations of the current study design. A larger, more heterogeneous sample from more than one institution coupled with a more rigorous design and developed instruments for capturing posthospital care of all participants will help elucidate the predictive capability of the DCSES. Such a method can also examine the possible response bias found in the current study. Although the numbers were small, the inpatient 2-year nonresponders were significantly more likely to be male and/or have a history or a current problem with alcohol (see Table 10.1). Second, a reliable and valid risk profile would be useful in guiding dismissal and follow-up plans for patients and providers. Clinical nursing case management and/or other models of care might be useful resources for patients being dismissed from a treatment program that are identified by the DCSES as at-risk for relapse. Targeting specific items rated low on the DCSES could be a focus of research. Additionally, more frequent follow-up assessment, coupled with teaching patients how to recognize their prodromal signs of depression, might result in earlier intervention and possible prevention of a major depressive episode. Further research may lead to new ways to increase self-efficacy in coping with depression, hopefully resulting in more effective coping and fewer episodes.

REFERENCES

American Psychiatric Association. (1994). *Diagnostic and statistical manual of mental disorders* (4th ed.). Washington, DC: Author.

Bandura, A. (1997). *Self-efficacy: The exercise of control.* New York: W. H. Freeman.

Bernier, M., & Avard, J. (1986). Self-efficacy, outcome, and attrition in a weight-reduction program. *Cognitive Therapy and Research, 10*(3), 319-338.

Condiotte, M. M., & Lichtenstein, E. (1981). Self-efficacy and relapse in smoking cessation programs. *Journal of Consulting and Clinical Psychology, 49*(5), 648-658.

Devons, G. M., Orme, C. M., Costello, G., Binik, Y. M., Frizzell, B., Stam, H. J., et al. (1988). Measuring depressive symptoms in illness populations: Psychometric properties of the Center for Epidemiologic Studies Depression (CES-D) scale. *Psychology & Health, 2,* 139-156.

Dolce, J. J. (1987). Self-efficacy and disability beliefs in behavioral treatment of pain. *Behaviour Research and Therapy, 25*(4), 289-299.

Doris, A., Ebmeier, K, & Shajahan, P. (1999). Depressive Illness. *Lancet, 354*(9187), 1369-1375.

Frank, E., Kupfer, D. J., Cornes, C., Jarrett, D. B., Mallinger, A. G., Thase, M. E., et al. (1990). Three-year outcomes for maintenance therapies in recurrent depression. *Archives of General Psychiatry, 47*(12), 1093-1099.

Kaplan, E., & Turkington, C. (1997). *What is depression?* Retrieved November 7, 2000, from http://my.webmd.com/content/dmk/dmk-article-5963098

Keller, M. B., & Boland, R. J. (1998). Implications of failing to achieve successful long-term maintenance treatment of recurrent unipolar major depression. *Biological Psychiatry, 44,* 348-360.

Kessler, R., C., McGonagle, K. A., Zhao, S., Nelson, C. B., Hughes, M., Eshleman, S., Wittchen, H., & Kendler, K. (1994). Lifetime and 12-month prevalence of DSM-III-R psychiatric disorders in the United States: Results from the national comorbidity survey. *Archives of General Psychiatry, 51*(1), 8-29.

Kessler, R., C., Zhao, S., Blazer, D. G., & Swartz, M. (1997). Prevalence, correlates, and course of minor depression and major depression in the national comorbidity survey. *Journal of Affective Disorders, 45,* 19-30.

Kluiter, H., Giel, R., Nienhuis, E. J., Ruphan, M., & Wiersma, D. (1992). Predicting feasibility of day treatment for unselected patients referred for inpatient psychiatric treatment: Results of a randomized trial. *American Journal of Psychiatry, 149*(9), 1199-1205.

Lin, E. H. B., Katon, W. J., Von Korff, M., Russo, J. E., Simon, G. E., Bush, T. M., et al. (1998). Relapse of depression in primary care: Rate and clinical predictors. *Archives of Family Medicine, 7*(5), 443-449.

National Institute of Mental Health. (2000). *The invisible disease.* Retrieved November 7, 2000, from http://www.nimh.nih.gov/publicat/invisible.cfm

Perraud, S. (2000). Development of the depression coping self-efficacy scale (DCSES). *Archives of Psychiatric Nursing, 14*(6), 276-284.

Quiring, J. M., Monroe, S. M., Simons, A. D., & Thase, M. E. (2002). Does early intervention increase latency to relapse in major depressive disorder?: Re-evaluation with cognitive behavior therapy. *Journal of Affective Disorders, 70*(1), 155-163.

Simon, G. E., Von Korff, M., Ludman, E. J., Katon, W. J., Rutter, C., Unutzer, J., et al. (2002). Cost-effectiveness of a program to prevent depression relapse in primary care. *Medical Care, 40*(10), 941-950.

Sullivan, M. D., LaCroix, A. Z., Russo, J., & Katon, W. J. (1998). Self-efficacy and self-reported functional status in coronary heart disease: A six-month prospective study. *Psychosomatic Medicine, 60,* 473-478.

Tucker, S., Brust, S., & Richardson, S. (2002). Validity of the Depression Coping Self-Efficacy Scale. *Archives of Psychiatric Nursing, 16*(3), 125-133.

Weissman, M., Roger, C., Bland, M., Canino, G., Faravelli, C., Greenwald, S., et al. (1996). Cross-national epidemiology of major depression and bipolar disorder. *Journal of the American Medical Association, 276,* 293-299.